MASTER
THE HIP HINGE

The pre-cursor to the Deadlift, Bent-over Row, and Kettlebell Swing.

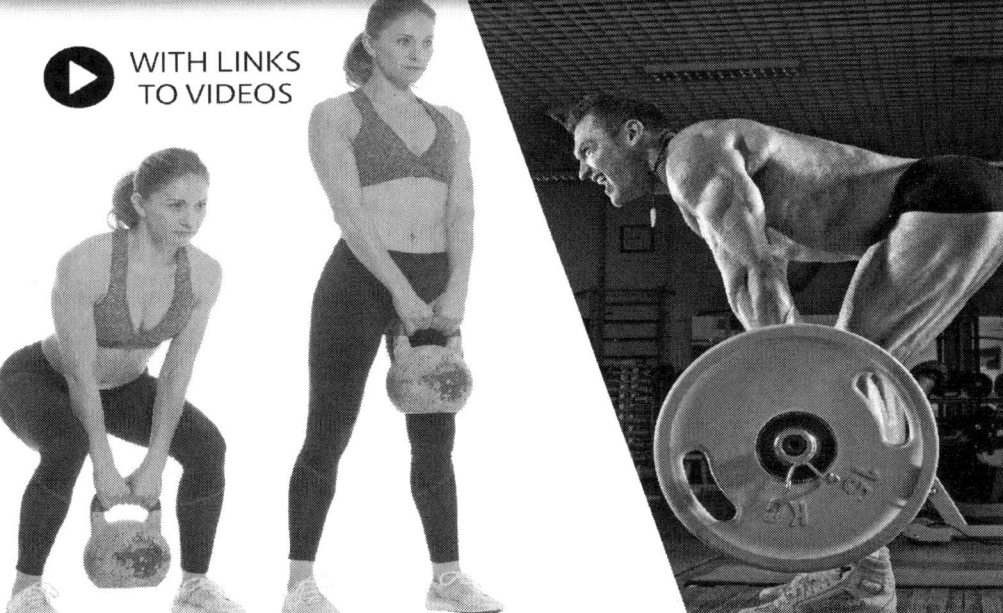

WITH LINKS
TO VIDEOS

By Taco Fleur
Cavemantraining.com

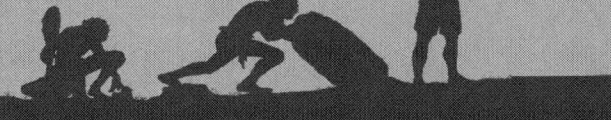

This book covers every intricate detail of the hip hinge movement, explained and broken down in such a way that everyone can understand it, it's basic but at the same time advanced.

Hip Hinge Movement—The Foundation For Swings, Deadlifts, Cleans, And More

Explained in plain English so everyone can understand it.

"The hip hinge is one of the fundamental movement patterns for human beings and Taco Fleur has provided a guide to help the reader own the movement. Broken down into component parts, with definitions and videos, this ebook is big on performing the hip hinge correctly. It is sure to become a valuable addition to your reference library."

*~ **Wendy Chappell***

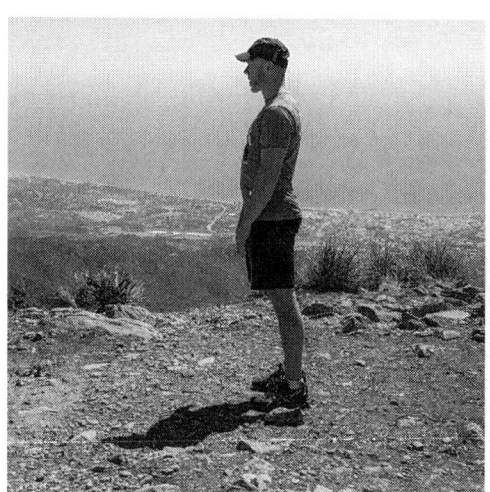 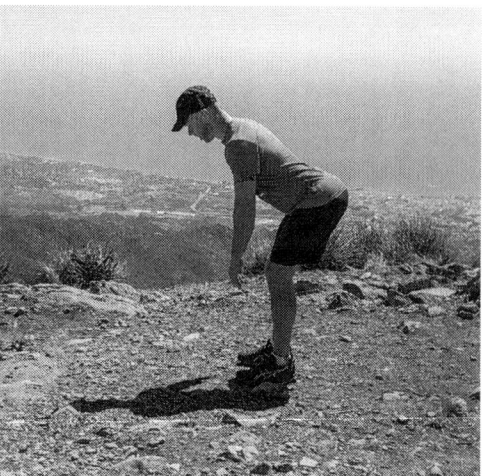

"This publication is a great asset for fitness enthusiasts. It covers an under-appreciated yet vital element in functional movement, the hip hinge. I'm glad I got the opportunity to help contribute to this important topic. I hope you find it useful and informative and, most importantly, incorporate this valuable information into your fitness routine."~

Derek Fronczak

(NESTA Certified Personal Fitness Trainer and Functional Training specialist)

The hip hinge is a fundamental movement in exercise. It is vital because knowing and performing it correctly will not only prevent injury but will allow you to work a large portion of the posterior chain muscles with a single movement. Also, a lot of important exercises—such as the kettlebell swing, the traditional deadlift, bent-over rows, cleans, and many more—depend on this movement.

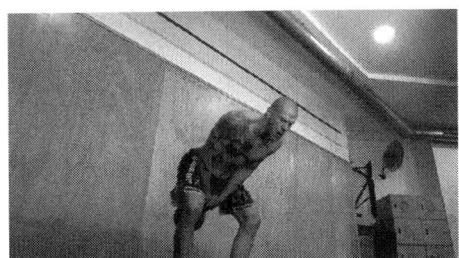 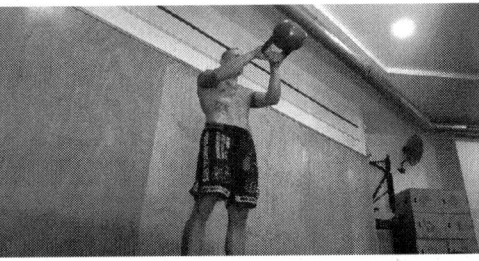

Master The Hip Hinge

About the Author

My name is Taco Fleur, and I'm an IKFF Certified Kettlebell Trainer, Russian Girevoy Sport Institute Kettlebell Coach, Kettlebell Level 1 + 2 Trainer, Kettlebell Science and Application, CrossFit Level 1 Trainer, MMA Conditioning Level 1, Kettlebell Sport Rank 2, MMA Fitness Level 1 + 2, Punchfit Trainer and Plyometrics Trainer Certified, with a purple belt in Brazilian Jiu-Jitsu. I have owned and set-up 3 functional kettlebell gyms in Australia and Vietnam, and lived in the Netherlands, Australia, Vietnam, and Thailand. I'm currently living in Spain.

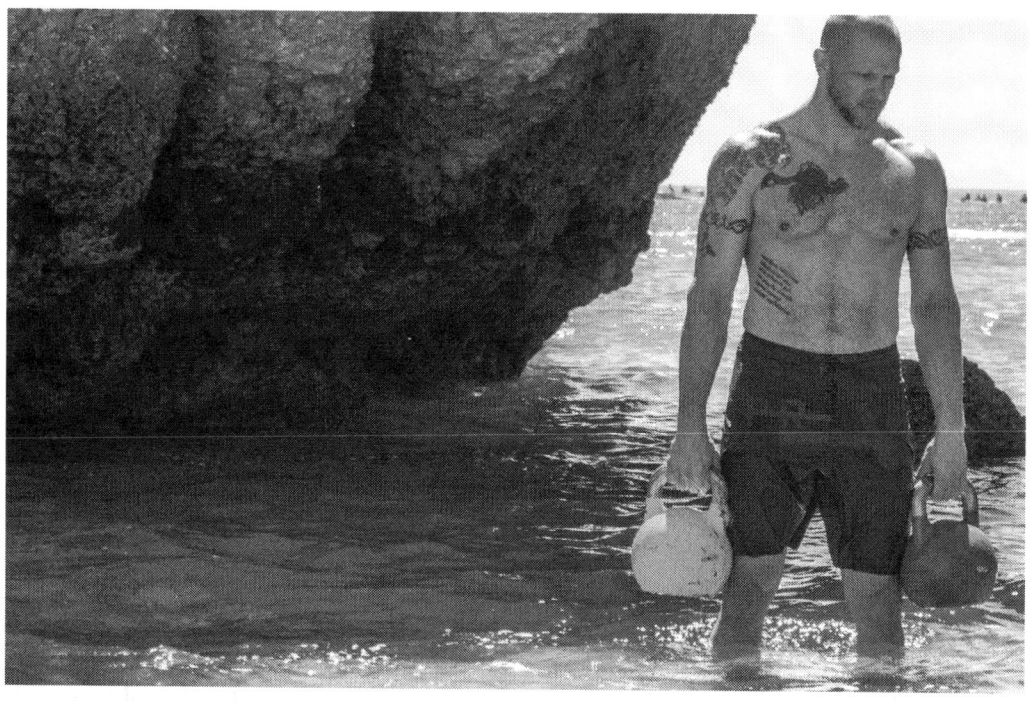

The first thing I'd like you to know about me is that I do **not** know everything, I don't pretend to know everything, and I never will. I'm on a path of life-long learning. I believe there is always something to learn from someone, no matter who they are. I've been physically active since the day I arrived on this earth in 1973. I got serious about training in 1999, touched a kettlebell for the first time in 2004, and got serious about kettlebell training in 2009. I'm here to do what I love most, and that is to share my knowledge with the world.

Some of my personal bests are 400 burpees performed in under one hour; 500 kettlebell snatches, 500 swings and 500 double-unders all completed in one session; 250 alternating dead clean and presses in one session with 20kg; 200 pull-ups in one session; 200 unbroken kettlebell swings with a 28kg; most kettlebell swings completed in one session with a 28kg (1,501); most total kettlebell swings done in 28 days with a 28kg (11,111);windmill with a 40kg kettlebell; lugged a kettlebell up a 1,184m mountain; 160kg dead lift; 250 alternating dead clean and presses in one session with 20kg; 100 snatches on sand with a 24kg kettlebell; 300 unbroken clean and jerk with 20kg/44lbs; 85kg Olympic Squat Snatch; Gold medalist with 30 minutes of unbroken 16kg half snatches for a total of 532 reps; and one of my favorites is lugging the first kettlebell up the highest mountain in mainland Spain 3,479m/11,414f with 16kg. I mention these PBs not to boast but to demonstrate that I have a good understanding of technique and movement across different areas. This demonstrates especially with the high reps, an area in which most commonly tearing of the hands occurs.

My own training and goals are geared around GPP (General Physical Preparedness) which involves kettlebell training, calisthenics, and CrossFit. I like high-volume reps but also like greasing the groove now and again. My main goals are to remains as agile as possible, remain mobile, train in as many planes of movements as possible, and learn as many different exercise combinations and movements as possible while having fun and enjoying Brazilian Jiu Jitsu. I'm no Arnold Schwarzenegger and never will be, but strength is not solely defined by physical appearance and huge bulging muscles.

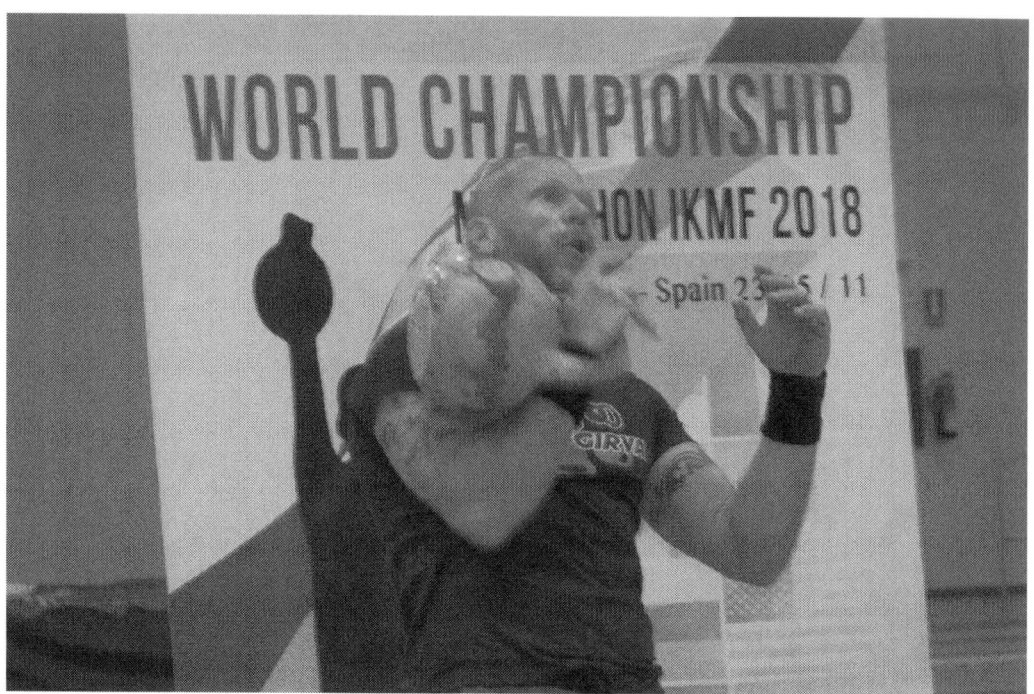

You can read more about my training, philosophy, and other ramblings on my website, www.cavemantraining.com, and on my YouTube channel, bit.ly/youtube-cavemantraining, which at the time of writing has over 34,000 subscribers and more than 6 million views.

SUBSCRIBE

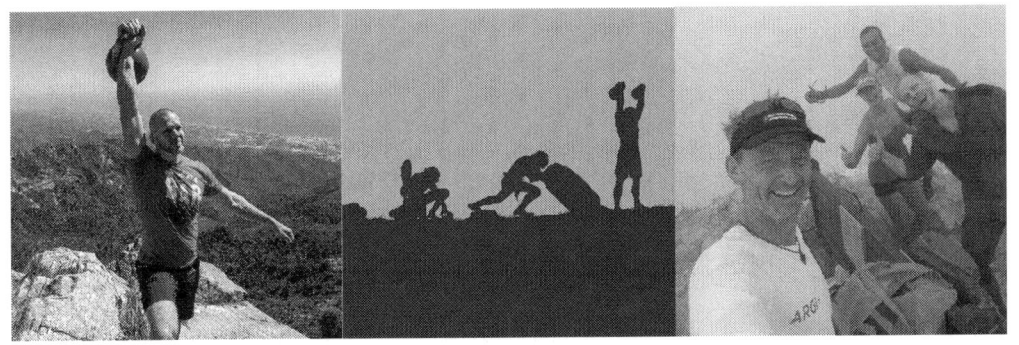

Add me: Facebook.com/taco.fleur or Facebook.com/coach.taco.fleur

Facebook.com/Cavemantraining or Facebook.com/Cavemantraining.Magazine
for up-to-date articles and news.

Please note that this material may not be reproduced or publicized elsewhere without the written consent of the author me@tacofleur.com.

If you bought this as a PDF/electronic copy, note that it is digitally signed and password protected with identifiable information.

Kettlebell training is my passion and expertise, hence the reason I choose to write about the hip hinge first, the hip hinge is one of the most important movements to learn before moving on to cleaning, swinging or snatching a kettlebell. Furthermore, I also love to deadlift, again, the hip hinge is the movement on which the conventional deadlift is based.

Following are the books published by Cavemantraining:

- **Master The Hip Hinge**
  On Amazon, iTunes, or Cavemantraining

- **Master The Lunge**
  On Amazon, iTunes, or Cavemantraining

- **Master Kettlebell Grips**
  On Amazon, iTunes, or Cavemantraining

- **Kettlebell Training Fundamentals**
  On Amazon, iTunes, or Cavemantraining
  Contains the kettlebell grips and racking book

- **Snatch Physics**
  On Amazon, iTunes, or Cavemantraining

- **Master The Kettlebell Clean**
  On Amazon, iTunes, or Cavemantraining

- **Master The Kettlebell Press**
  On Amazon or Cavemantraining

- **Master The Kettlebell Swing**
  On Amazon or Cavemantraining

- **Kettlebell Workouts And Challenges 1.0**
  On Amazon, iTunes, or Cavemantraining

- **Flexibility, Mobility, and Strength Without Yoga**

  On Amazon, iTunes, or Cavemantraining

- And more on Cavemantraining

This is version *five* of the book, originally written December 2015 and last updated in April 2019. This book is a continuous work in progress, with additional content added as it becomes available. You can stay up-to-date on the most recent version just by liking our Cavemantraining Facebook page. To receive a **free copy of updated versions** in the future please leave your email on the following link http://eepurl.com/dfC-8L.

While writing this book my objective was to cover as many basic and intrinsic details of the hip hinge as possible. I know people learn and understand things in different ways; I've therefore done my best to present some of the same information in a different style, or with different explanations.

I can highly recommend to perform the movements as explained (where possible and safe) while you read this book, this will provide you with a better understanding, and there will also be a higher retention rate of information.

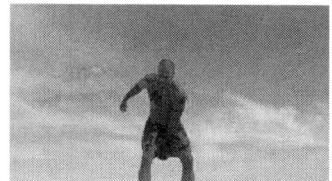 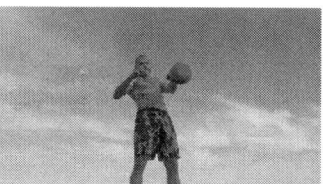 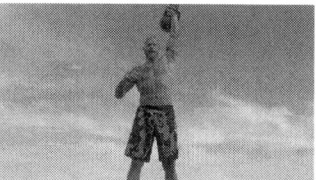

Hip hinge for the kettlebell snatch.

Disclaimer

This is a book, not a personal training session, I don't know your skills, injuries, training environment, training experience or anything else about you. The information contained in this book is based on my knowledge and experience — you alone need to make the decision whether this knowledge works for you, whether a certain exercise is safe for you, whether a program is safe for you. Only you (and you alone) can make that decision unless you employ a local trainer, or work with me online. If you have current or past injuries I recommend you to get a professional opinion on whether the hip hinge is safe for you.

With that said, I'm always more than happy to volunteer some of my time, and try to answer simple questions in moderation on *Facebook.com/cavemantraining*

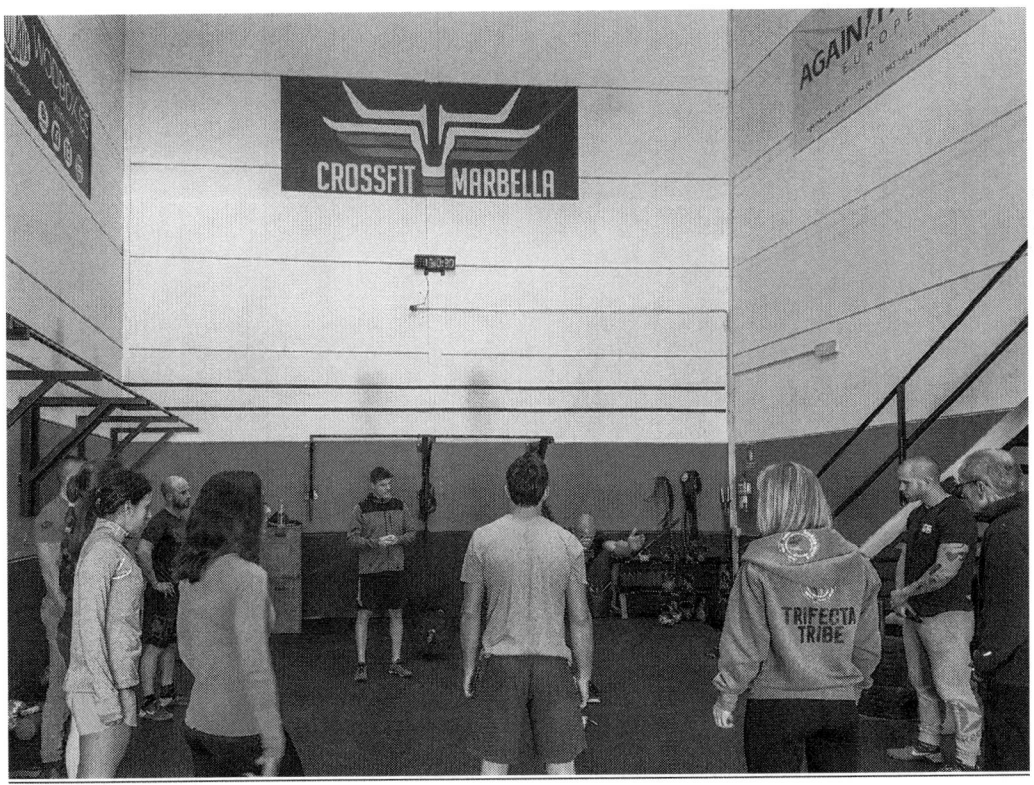

Table of Contents

Who Is This Book For?

This book is for Crossfitters, fitness enthusiasts, for anyone that wants to understand and properly perform the foundation for deadlifts, swings, bent-over rows, and cleans; anyone that wants to lift safely in their day-to-day life; and anyone wanting to regain their mobility.

What Will You Learn?

After reading this book you will understand, how to perform the hip hinge safely; avoid pains; how to use it for exercise; what muscles are used; find faults; provide corrections; and how to cue the movement to your students.

Definitions

Probably the most boring bit of this book, but if you don't understand the definitions, you won't understand certain parts of the book. It's only a few, so invest some time to fully understand them:

- **Flex / flexion** = contraction; shortening the muscle.

- **Extend / extension** = to bring outwards; if your arm was hanging and you would extend your arm to shake someone's hand, that would be arm extension – returning the arm to full extension after a bicep curl would be extension, lengthening the muscle.

- **Isotonic** = taking place with normal contraction (isos = equal, tonos = tone) – a muscular contraction in which the length of the muscle changes.

- **Eccentric** = an isotonic contraction where the muscle lengthens.

- **Concentric** = an isotonic contraction where the muscle shortens.

- **Isometric** = having equal dimensions (isos = equal, metria = measuring); a muscular contraction in which the length of the muscle does not change.

- **Core** = in the context of this book the abdominals, obliques, erector spinae and surrounding musculature.

- **Anterior** = front.

- **Posterior** = back.

- **Resistance** = the impeding or stopping effect exerted by one object on another (resistance training).

- **Neutral spine** = the natural position of the spine when all 3 curves of the spine (thoracic, lumbar, sacral) are present and in good alignment.

- **Thoracic spine** = the upper- and middle-back.

- **Laterally** = at, towards, or from the side or sides; sideways.

- **Bilaterally** = something has two sides or affects both sides of something.
- **Proprioception** = the sense of the relative position of neighboring parts of the body and strength of effort being employed in movement.

- **ROM** = range of motion.

- **AKA** = also known as.

- **Prime mover** = muscles that initiate the source of movement.
- **Agonist** = a muscle whose contraction moves a part of the body directly.
- **Antagonist** = a muscle whose action counteracts that of another specified muscle.

Master The Hip Hinge

Author *Taco Fleur*

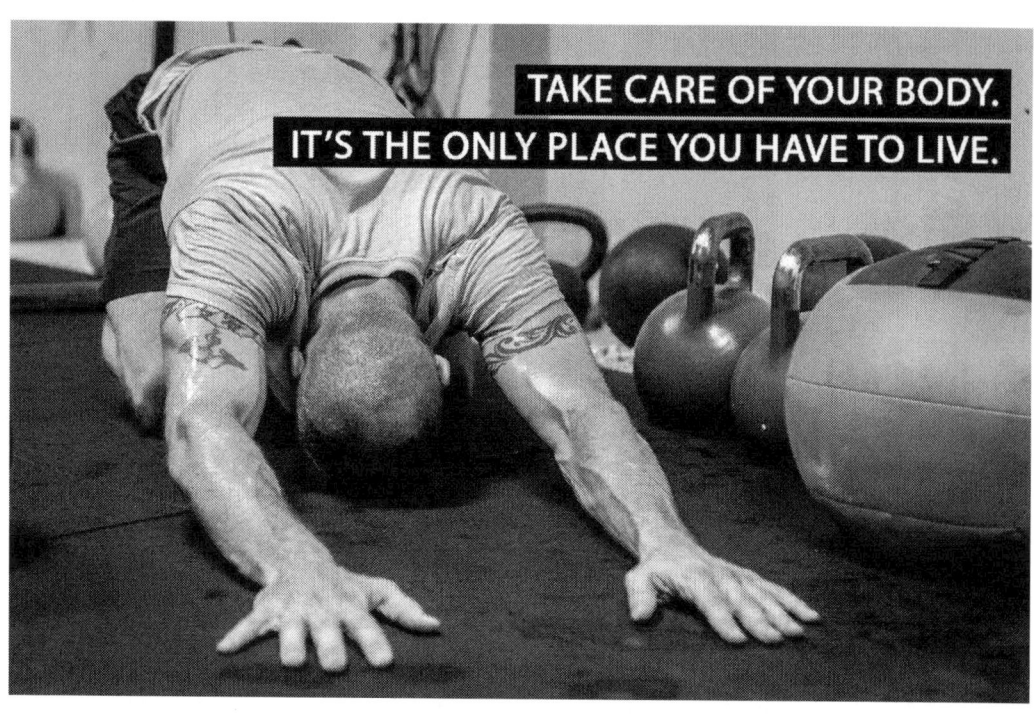

Master The Hip Hinge

What Is It?

The hip hinge consists of two parts: a break at the hips, allowing the torso to come forward and down (flexion); the reverse, where the torso comes back into upright position (extension). A complete hip hinge is flexion and extension of the hips.

What Is It Not?

The hip hinge is not a squat. This is very important to know as this is the most common mistake people make when trying to perform the hip hinge movement. Yes, the squat contains a hinge at the hips, but the hip hinge does not contain a squat (flexing three joints).

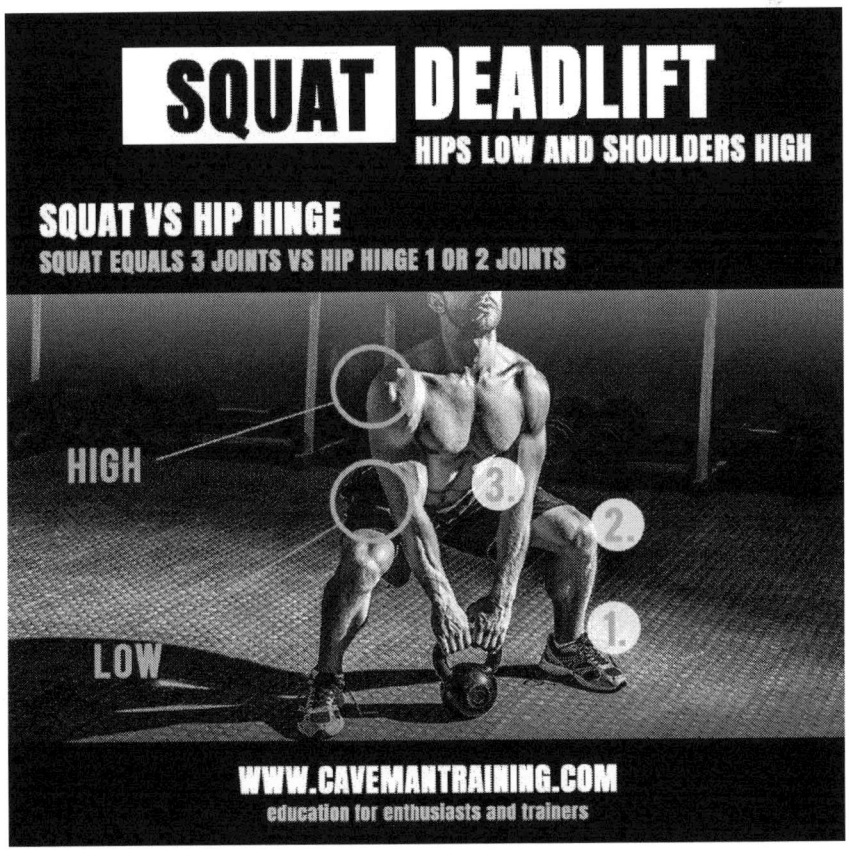

A squat movement contains a hip hinge movement.

Master The Hip Hinge

Quick Comparison

A quick comparison between the hip hinge and squat:

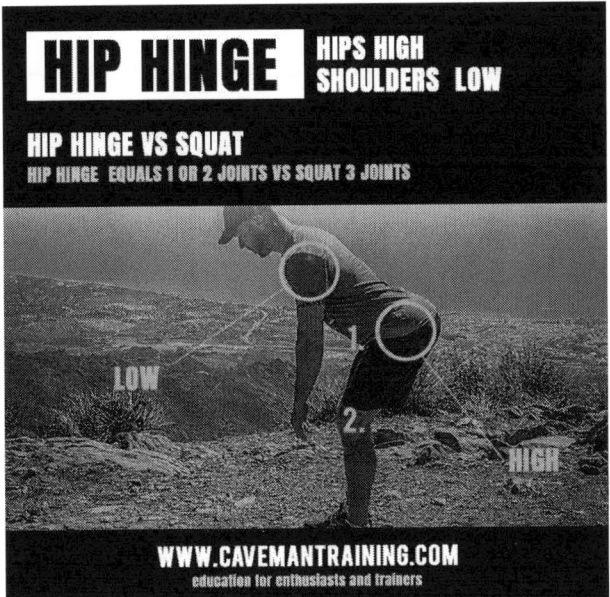

Objective: Shoulders lower to the ground.

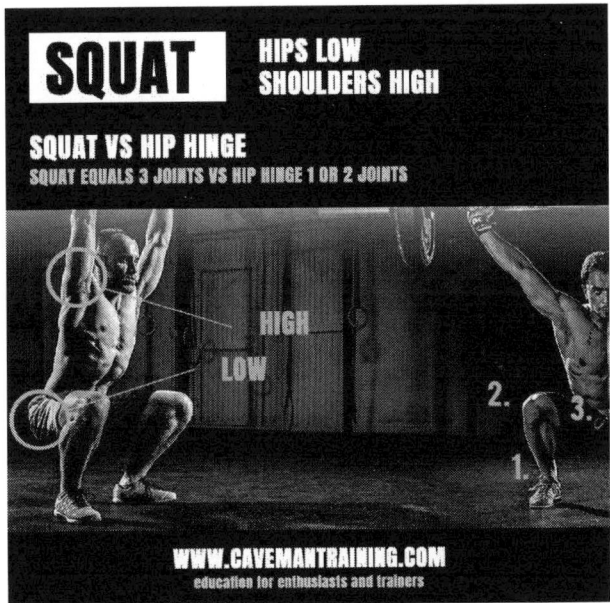

Objective: Hips lower to the ground.

Objective

The objectives of a hip hinge can be:

- To put load on the gluteus maximus and hamstrings for strength purposes. This is achieved by bringing the shoulders towards the ground with a neutrally aligned spine. Especially with added weight.
- To put load on the erector spinae (back) for strength purposes.
- To work on flexibility. This is achieved by working on maximum range.
- To pick up an object.

Confusion

The hip hinge is often referred to by people—even many long time trainers—as a "deadlift". This is due to the conventional deadlift being a hip hinge movement, and this version is the one most often seen and used; however, a deadlift can also be performed with a squatting motion—put simply, a deadlift is **not always** performed with a hip hinge. A couple of deadlift variations are: Suitcase deadlift, sumo squat deadlift, staggered kettlebell deadlift, lunge deadlift, and so on.

Furthermore, *hip hinge* describes the **movement** pattern, and *deadlift* describes the **range** (from "dead" to "lift"). To give you another example of range "hang lift", describes the range from hanging to lift. To lift means, to raise to a higher position or level.

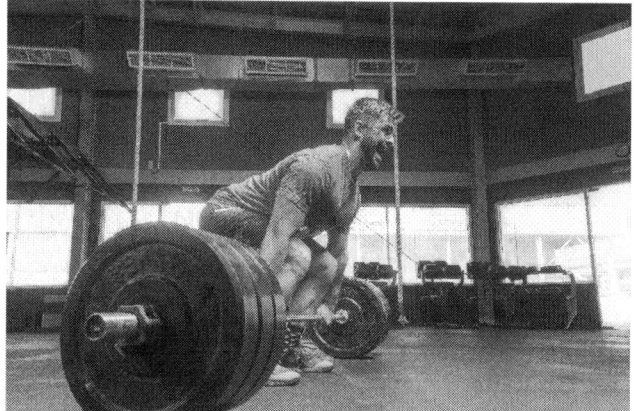

Deadlift.

Another major reason for confusion is because popular websites like Wikipedia do not correctly name the type of deadlift they're covering. This can be seen here: https://en.wikipedia.org/wiki/Deadlift. The deadlift illustrated is the hip hinge deadlift, AKA the conventional deadlift, and nowhere do they mention the squat deadlift, thus making people think that a deadlift can only ever be a hip hinge.

Dead = not moving

Lift = raise to a higher position or level

Daily Life Applications

Here are some examples of when the hip hinge is used in daily life:

- At the basin drinking water or washing your face
- Reaching for something over the table
- Picking up light objects from a dresser
- Picking up groceries

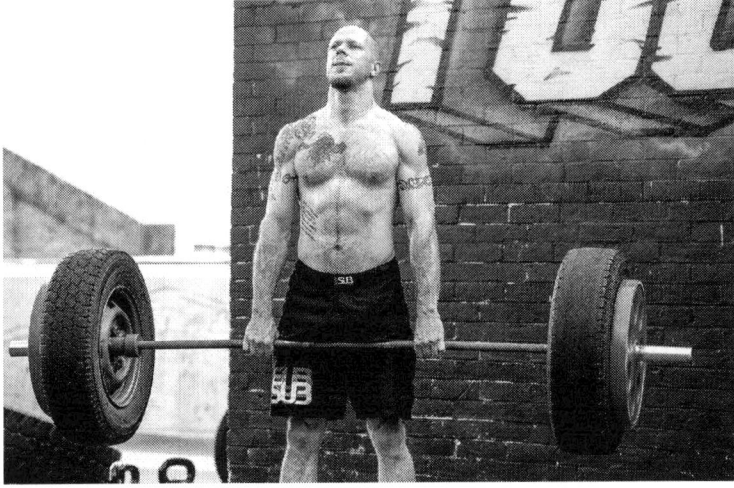

Exercise Applications

Here are some examples of when the hip hinge is used in exercise:

- Deadlift (hip hinge style)
- CrossFit Barbell Clean

  Although this has changed since I wrote this book in 2015 and now, the official CrossFit YouTube channel demonstrates a clear hip hinge https://youtu.be/EKRiW9Yt3Ps but in the boxes I've trained it is turning more into a squat with the knees coming forward and the shoulders higher. The squat movement is to be able to safely lift heavier weight.

- Bent-Over Row
- Conventional Kettlebell Swing and American Kettlebell Swing in CrossFit
- Good Morning
- Cable Pull-Through
- Battling Ropes

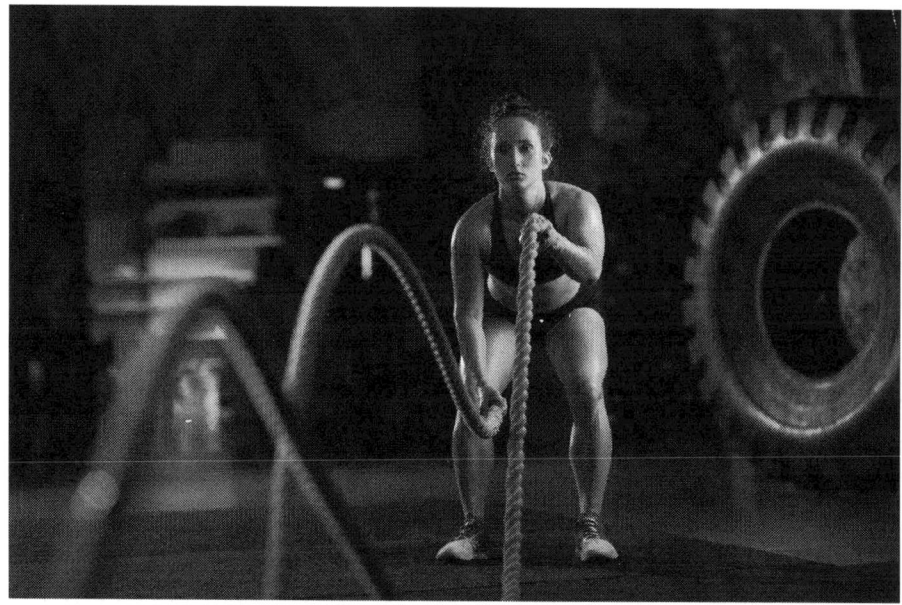

Battling Ropes.

Requirements

Not everybody can perform a good hip hinge straight away, and it's not always because they don't understand the movement. There are requirements one must meet before being able to do a perfectly executed hip hinge, namely: core, gluteus maximus, and calf strength, and hamstring flexibility.

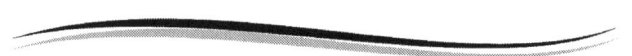

What Are Hips?

The hips are a projection of the pelvis and upper thighbone on each side of the body in human beings.

🛈 Projection refers to anything that extends outwards from something else; in this case the upper thighbone (femur) projects from the pelvis.

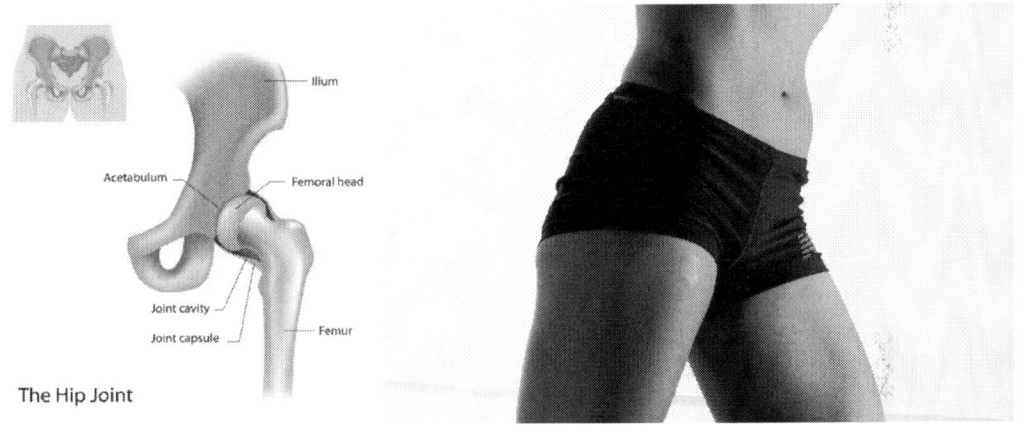

The Hip Joint

What Is a Hinge?

The hinge in general terms is a movable joint or mechanism on which a door, gate, or lid swings as it opens and closes or which connects linked objects. In the case of humans, and relevant to the topic at hand, the hinge is located between the upper body and lower body.

Google definition: a natural joint which performs a function similar to that of a man-made hinge, for example that of a bivalve shell; a movable joint or mechanism on which a door, gate, or lid swings as it opens and closes or which connects linked objects.

Merriam-Webster definition: a flexible ligamentous joint; a jointed or flexible device on which a door, lid, or other swinging part turns.

Wikipedia definition: In biology, many joints function as hinges like the elbow joint.

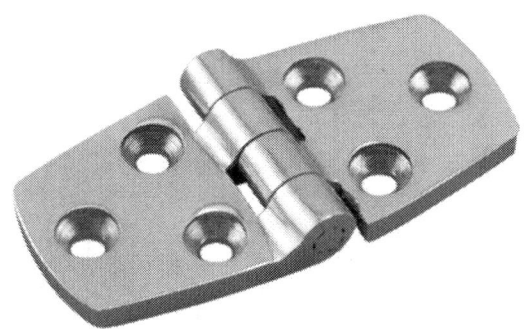

Cavemantraining Definition of the Hip Hinge

Movement
- Shoulders moving toward the ground
- Hips remaining in place or moving back and slightly down

Joints
- Fixed: hips
- Variable: knees

A hip hinge is performed in standing position, with the objective being to move the torso toward horizontal, this is achieved through flexion in the hip joints. The movement can also be accompanied by flexion in a second joint, that of the knees, which is cause for the hips to move back and down. The function of added knee flexion is to create a more balanced weight distribution, especially with weighted hip hinges like deadlifts. If the ankle joints move and dorsiflexion is achieved, the definition of the movement changes to a squat.

The objective of the hip hinge exercise is to tax the gluteus maximus and hamstrings (hip extensors). A completely horizontal torso provides the maximum resistance for the hip flexors, and the more it moves towards vertical, the more resistance is removed.

The maximum recommend hip flexion in general is 45° for weighted hip hinges.

Even though the most popular hip movement is called the hip hinge, the hip joints are not a hinge joint but a ball and socket (spheroid) joint.

The knees, ankles and elbows are hinge joints.

The joints found between the phalanges of the fingers and toes are hinge joints.

A hip hinge is a hip hinge (1 or 2 joints), a squat is a squat, even though a squat has a hip hinge in it, it's still a squat (three joints), just like a burpee contains a plank but is still a burpee.

Posterior Chain

The posterior chain is a group of muscles on the posterior (back) of the body. Examples of these muscles include but are not limited to: the biceps femoris (part of your hamstrings), gluteus maximus, erector spinae muscle group, trapezius, and posterior deltoids.

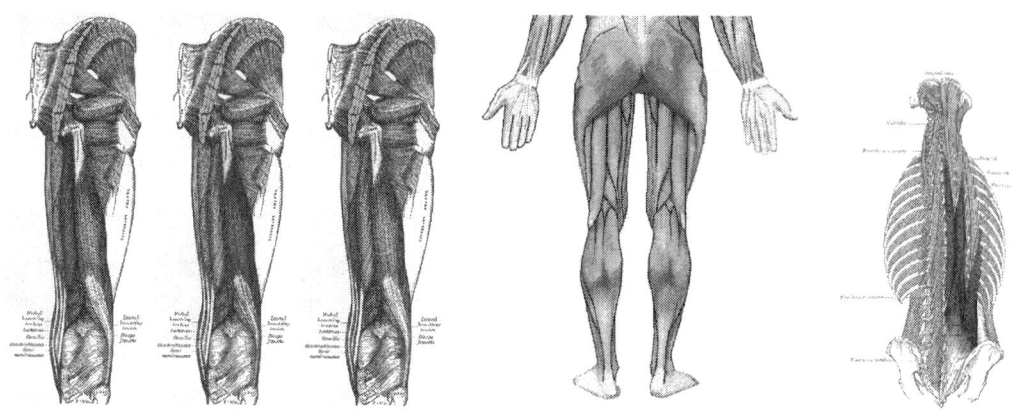

Resistance

The hip hinge movement can be performed with bodyweight or with added resistance, such as a kettlebell, barbell, sandbag, etc.

More muscle groups are recruited once resistance is added, which means the upper body will need to do more work to keep the spine neutral, to keep the shoulders back and safely in their sockets.

One Or Two Joints?

The hip hinge can be performed with one or two joints, knees and/or hips, the knee joints are the variable. The reason for using the knee joints, and bringing the hips back is to create counterbalance, especially with weighted hip hinges. Removing the knee joints from the movement will allow you to isolate more, and put more focus on the gluteus maximus. However, performing stiff legged hip hinge deadlifts, or bodyweight hip hinges, is a progression, and should not be performed at the beginning of ones exercise journey. Consider them at the top end of your progressional journey.

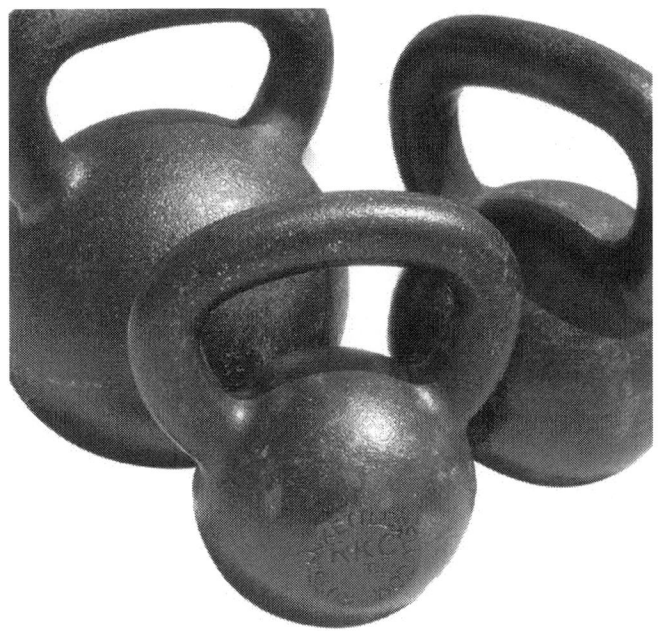

Dynamic vs Static

Dynamic hip hinges are those in which you're moving into flexion and extension upon each repetition, for example: deadlifts, kettlebell swings, Crossfit barbell cleans, etc. Static hip hinges are those where you're moving into flexion and remain there for several repetitions or duration of time, for example: Bent-over rows or *Uttanasana* (yoga pose). In static hip hinges you keep the gluteus maximus and other hip extensors in isometric contraction.

Muscles

To help you understand and remember the important muscles and muscle groups, below are some definitions and explanation of the more common recurring words:

- Femoris = thigh
- Brachii = arm
- Minimus = inner (not direct translation)
- Medial / medius = middle

- Maximus = outer (not direct translation)
- Bi = two
- Tri = three
- Quadri = four
- Cep = head (bicep, tricep, quadricep)
- Rectus = straight

For example, in the name *Biceps Femoris*, the last part of the name will tell you that the muscle is located in the lower part of the body, in particular the thigh. The same applies to Rectus **Femoris**, Quadriceps **Femoris,** etc.

Muscle Groups Worked

When explaining exercises, programming, for yourself or others, it's important to know what muscles or muscle groups are worked to be able to choose correctly targeted exercises, and explain what muscles to activate (i.e. contract and relax).

It can become extremely complex when covering muscles, and muscle groups involved with any exercise. In reality, almost every muscle in your body is used in some way when performing any exercise, even if only in a supportive isometric contraction.

To keep things basic and understandable, **focus on the primary movers**, the main muscle group(s) targeted with any exercise (i.e. the muscle we want to strengthen and the one that drives the movement). The other muscles are used for assistance in the movement or for keeping the body stabilized. To give you an example not related to the hip hinge, think of chin-ups, they target the biceps/brachialis/brachioradialis, but also involves the delts, lats and other muscles.

Muscle groups are not just one muscle, but a set of muscles.

Below are the main muscle groups you should learn and understand. Underneath these are listed those that are complimentarily involved (i.e. synergists and stabilizers).

Master The Hip Hinge   *Author Taco Fleur*

Main Muscle Targets

The main targets of the hip hinge movement are the **gluteus maximus** (the biggest part of the glutes), biceps femoris (long head/part of hamstrings), semitendinosus (part of hamstrings), semimembranosus (part of hamstrings), and adductor magnus. These muscles are also known as the hip extensors. Your hip flexors also play a roll in the hip hinge, however, the hip flexors are the ones you'll really feel and work. The hip flexors pull the hips down and they are; psoas major, iliacus, tensor fasciae latae, sartorius, and rectus femoris.

With added resistance, the core muscles should be included as main targets. The core muscles become an extremely important muscle group once resistance is added to this movement, and is heavily involved. One should have a relatively strong core before attempting to perform this movement with added weight.

🛈The hamstrings are the main muscles that receive dynamic stretching.

🛈The gluteus maximus, gluteus minimus, gluteus medius are collectively referred to as glutes (three muscles).

🛈The erector spinae muscle groups function to straighten the back and aids in spinal rotation. In the case of the hip hinge they act to prevent your torso from falling forward once the hips move back.

🛈In the case of the hip hinge, the hip flexor muscle groups are engaged when pulling yourself down into the hip hinge, if you simply fall into the hip hinge, the hip flexors will not actively be engaged.

Details

When performing any exercise it's important to be knowledgeable about the muscles involved for numerous reasons, the main ones being:

- To know what muscles to activate for the movement

- To know what muscles you're targeting (i.e. strengthening) with the exercise
- To know where you went wrong when experiencing pain

Another reason to have muscle awareness is for Mind-Muscle Connection (MMC); this is the ability to connect with the correct muscles during exercise, and contract or relax them appropriately. A great example of MMC (or temporary lack thereof) is the inability to connect and contract the gluteus maximus in a lot of people. Typically, poking or hitting the gluteus maximus with your fingers or fists will provide location awareness, and assist in the ability to connect this muscle with a given movement.

Muscles at the front of the body are used to flex, and muscles at the back to extend; in the case of the hip hinge, we use the hip flexors for hip flexion, and the hip extensors for hip extension. There are more muscles involved in the movement and stabilization, but these are the prime movers.

Hip flexors and hip extensors, are two muscle groups that can be referred to as an antagonist pair. They control a given movement, which means they oppose each other, as in they initiate, limit or regulate the movement, as one muscle set contracts, the other relaxes. As an example, if the hip extensors stayed contracted while the hip flexors try to create hip flexion, then flexion of the hips would not be possible; on the other hand, if there was absolutely no action from the hip extensors during flexion then the torso would just fall forward.

Flexion of the hip

Agonists   Iliopsoas, Tensor fasciae latae, Gluteus medius

Antagonists   Gluteus maximus, Gluteus medius

Extension of the hip

Agonists   Gluteus maximus, Gluteus medius

Antagonists   Iliopsoas, Tensor fasciae latae, Gluteus medius

The hip hinge movement is used for deadlifting, bent-over rows, kettlebell swings and most importantly, it's part of maintaining hip mobility i.e. being able to freely and easily move the hips, whether it's to pick something up, to sit down, squat, or other daily activities. Although the hip flexors are prime movers for flexion, the hip hinge can be performed with a falling descent which takes out the hip flexors all together, but the opposite—taking out the hip extensors—is not possible in a standing position.

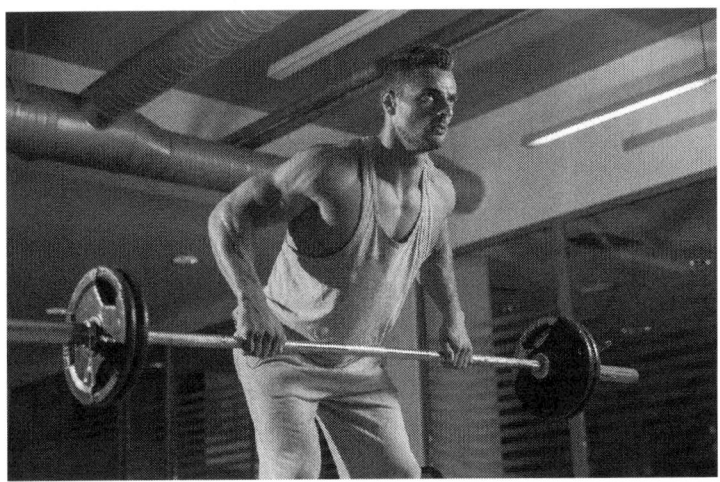

When it comes to muscles, it's also important to know the **origin** and **insertion** of the muscle. This will tell you what movement is initiated upon contraction of the muscle, i.e. what joint is being moved.

In brief, muscles are attached to bones on each end by tendons—the origin is the fixed attachment, and the insertion is the attachment that moves with contraction. For example: the biceps femoris long head has it's origin at your sit bone (ischial tuberosity) and the insertion is located at your shinbone, the lower part of your leg—there is more to it, but let's keep it simple.

Gluteal Muscle Group

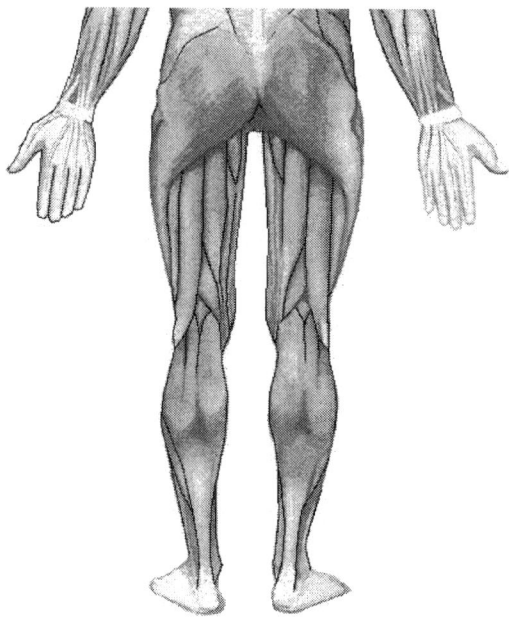

- Gluteus maximus
- Gluteus medius
- Gluteus minimus

Gluteus Maximus

The gluteus maximus top part (origin) of the muscle is connected to the ilium, the top of the pelvis. The bottom part (insertion) of the muscle is connected to the gluteal tuberosity, which is the ridge of the femur. The femur is the thigh bone; the bone in the top part of the leg.

From the gluteal muscles, only the gluteus maximus is a prime mover in the hip hinge, acting to extend the thigh at the hip. The other two gluteal muscles are involved with stabilization only, especially during one legged hip hinges. These two come a lot more in play with the squat during hip abduction.

Hamstring Muscle Group

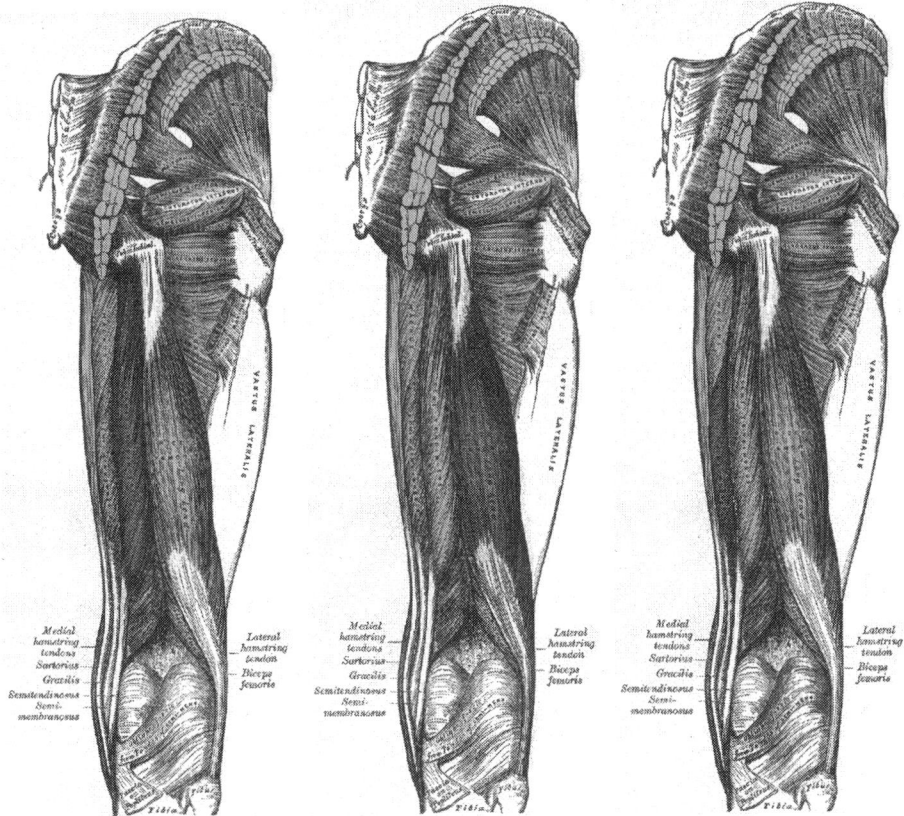

- Biceps femoris muscle
  - Long head
  - Short head
- Semitendinosus muscle
- Semimembranosus muscle

The hamstrings help to pull the hips back and down; thus, you should feel a stretch in the hamstrings when performing a conventional hip hinge with good form. A great way to visualize the action of the hamstrings is by standing on one leg and bringing the heel of the other leg towards the hips.

Try this simple action 10-20 times, making sure to keep the knee under or behind the hips if possible. Once you feel the activation of the hamstrings, you'll be aware of the action that their contraction provides.

Now imagine what happens with the same muscle contraction, but with your feet staying planted on the ground, you would pull the hips backwards, towards the heels. This is very important to understand, as this allows you to visualize exactly what the hamstrings do for you in the hip hinge—they can be activated to pull the hips back and down.

The hamstrings are also responsible for helping pull the pelvis upright, through muscle contraction which creates a pulling force at the bottom of the pelvis.

Semitendinosus Muscle (part of the hamstring muscle group)

The semitendinosus top part (origin) of the muscle is connected to the ischial tuberosity, AKA the sit bones located at the bottom of the hipbones. The bottom part (insertion) of the muscle is connected to the front of the bottom leg near the knee —also known as the shinbone— in medical terms known as the tibia.

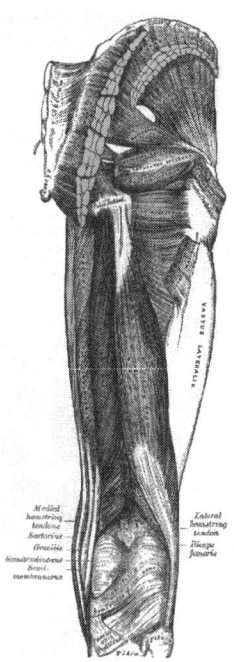

Semimembranosus Muscle (part of the hamstring muscle group)

The semimembranosus top part of the muscle is connected to the sit bones, the bottom of the hip bones. The bottom part of the muscle is connected to the back and inside of the bottom leg near the knee, to be more specific, it's connected to the medial condyle of the tibia, which is the round prominence at the end of the tibia bone.

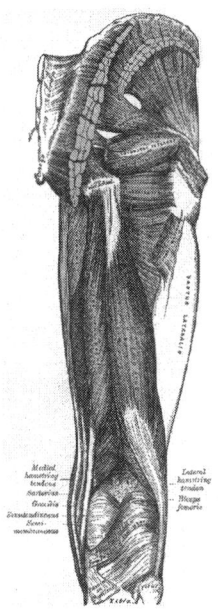

Biceps Femoris Muscle (part of the hamstring muscle group)

The biceps femoris consists of two heads, the long and the short head. The long head top part (origin) of the muscle is connected to the ischial tuberosity, AKA the sit bones, the bottom of the hip bones. The bottom part of the muscle is connected to the front of the fibula and lateral condyle of the tibia. The fibula or calf bone is a lower leg bone located on the lateral side of the tibia.

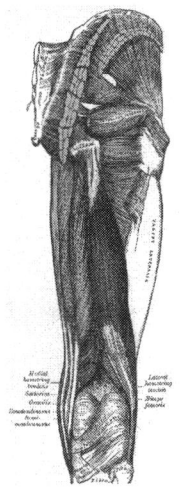

Master The Hip Hinge *Author Taco Fleur*

The short head top part of the muscle is connected lateral to the ridge of femur just past halfway of the bone. The bottom part of the muscle is connected to the head of the fibula and lateral condyle of the tibia.

Collectively these hamstrings work to extend the thigh (top leg) at the hip, flex the leg at the knee and medially rotate the leg if the knee is in a flexed state (bent). For visual reference: to perform extension of the thigh, stand on one leg and raise one knee up till almost inline with the hips, the part where your leg returns to standing is the extension, it's easier to imagine this with resistance provided, i.e. needing to push down (like walking up steps). Pull your heel towards the buttocks to action flexion of the knee.

🛈 The short head of the biceps femoris crosses only one joint (knee) and is therefore not involved in hip extension, but all other muscles from the hamstring group are.

Erector Spinae Muscles

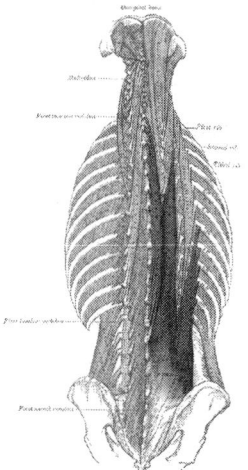

- Iliocostalis
  - ☐ Iliocostalis cervicis
  - ☐ Iliocostalis dorsi
  - ☐ Iliocostalis lumborum
- Longissimus
  - ☐ Longissimus thoracis

- ☐ Longissimus cervicis
- ☐ Longissimus capitis
- Spinalis
  - ☐ Spinalis dorsi
  - ☐ Spinalis cervicis
  - ☐ Spinalis capitis

More information about the erector spinae will be covered under the section *Back Aches and Pains*.

Hip Flexors

The hip flexors are used to create hip flexion—a good example of this is to bring your knee to your chest while standing. As mentioned, one can create hip flexion without the prime movers, simply by creating an angle at which the torso falls forward; however, actual pulling is required for rapid or controlled hip flexion, and thus actions involvement of the prime movers.

The hip flexors are (in descending order of importance to the action of flexing the hip joint):

- Collectively known as the iliopsoas or inner hip muscles:
  - ☐ Psoas major
  - ☐ Iliacus muscle
- Anterior compartment of thigh
  - ☐ Rectus femoris (part of the quadriceps muscle group)
  - ☐ Sartorius
- One of the gluteal muscles:
  - ☐ Tensor fasciae latae
- Medial compartment of thigh
  - ☐ Pectineus
  - ☐ Adductor longus
  - ☐ Adductor brevis
  - ☐ Gracilis

Master The Hip Hinge

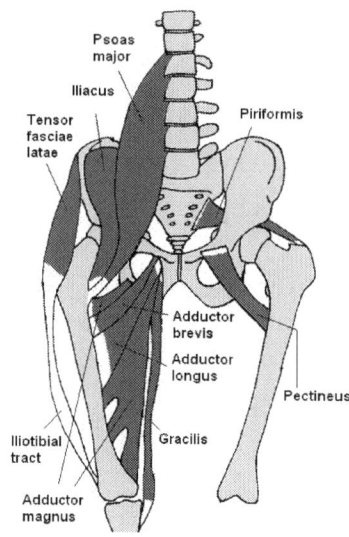

Hip Extensors

Hip extensors are the gluteus maximus, adductor magnus, and all muscles from the hamstring group except the short head of the biceps femoris.

The Hip Hinge Four Phase Movement Pattern

There is a **neutral, down, hang** and **up** phase to this movement.

Standing is the **neutral** phase

Moving down is the **down** phase

Reaching the bottom position is the **hang** phase

Moving up is the **up** phase

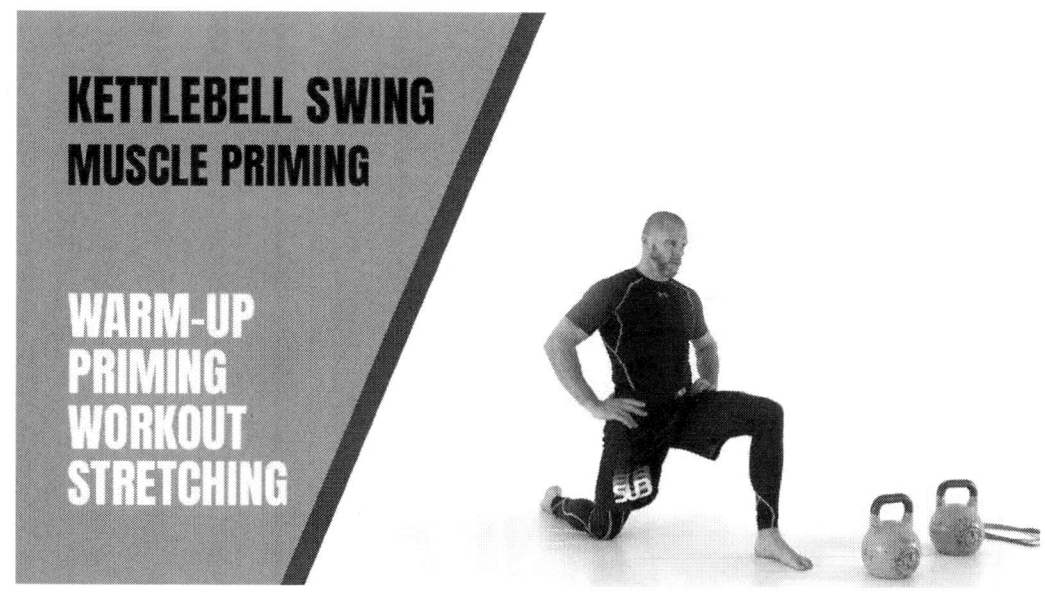

Caveman Kettlebell Swing Muscle Priming Routine

Whether you're new to the kettlebell swing or a seasoned athlete, a good routine for warming up and priming the muscles is gold. This is it.

Video https://go.cavemantraining.com/mthh-vid7

Warm-up

The first part of the warm-up is simple and focuses on getting the hips going and warming up the body.

- 5 single leg hip circles (each side)

- 10 jumping jacks

Repeat 6 times

Approx. 3 minutes

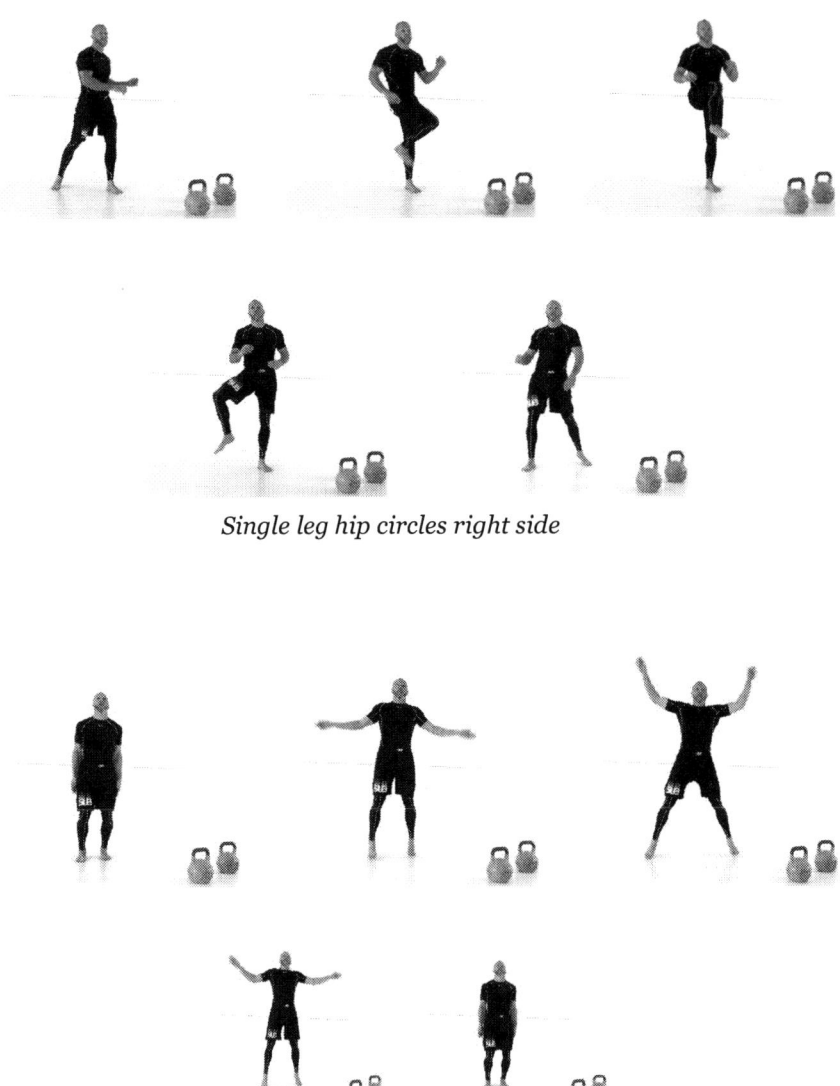

Single leg hip circles right side

The second part of the warm-up focusses on the hips plus posterior chain.

- Prone hip and thoracic hyperextension into pike

- Runners lunge (each side)

- Stand up

Repeat 6 times
Approx. 1 ½ minutes

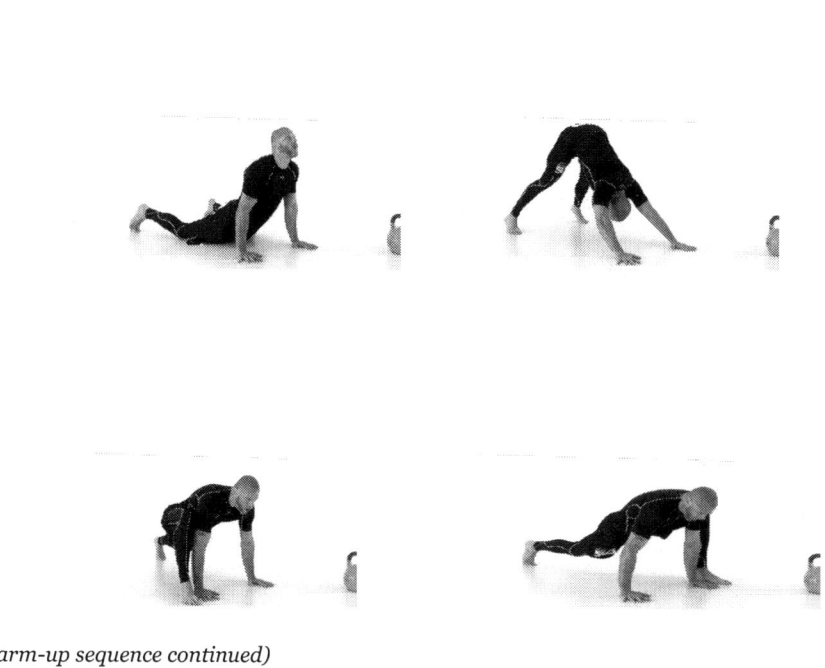

(warm-up sequence continued)

- Prone hip and thoracic hyperextension into pike

- Runners lunge and twist (each side)

- Stand up into arms overhead

Repeat 6 times

Approx. 2 minutes

Repeat the warm-up twice.

Approx. 10 minutes

Warning

Hip and thoracic hyperextension should be approached like anything, with progression and care. These two areas are usually not conditioned with the average person, this does not mean it's an area that should not be worked, it means it should be worked and progressed safely. Before you attempt this make sure you understand how to protect your lumbar and create range in with the hips and thoracic.

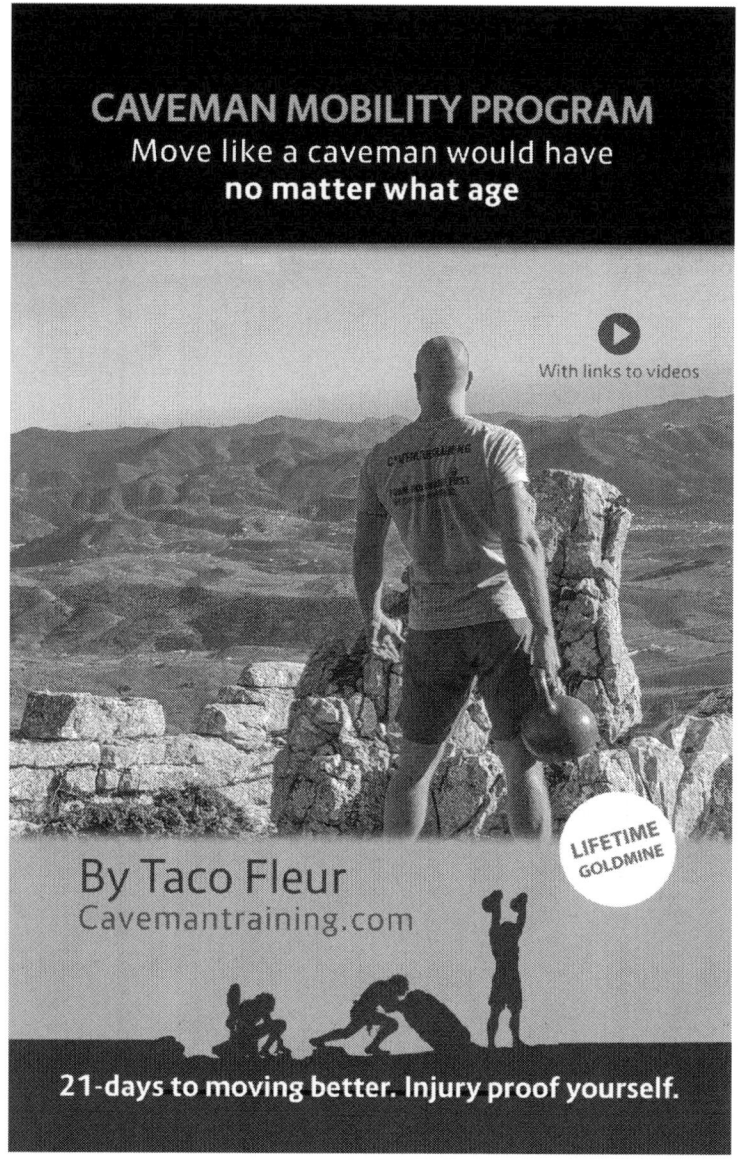

If in doubt, join our free Facebook groups and ask,
or buy the book on Amazon or Cavemantraining.

https://www.facebook.com/groups/unconventional.training/

Muscle priming

This is the part where you're connecting with the areas that are going to do the work for you.

The sequence is as follows:

- 5 x prone single leg hip hyperextensions (each side)
- 5 x prone thoracic hyperextensions
- 5 x kneeling hip extensions
- Kneeling lunge 10 x pulse (each side)
- 5 x true hip hinge
- 5 x quarter squat

Repeat twice
Approx. 4 minutes

Follow up with some shoulder circles to get the upper body loose.

1) Single leg hip hyperextensions

These are to connect with the gluteus maximus and feel the area which is going to do the primary work for you during swings.

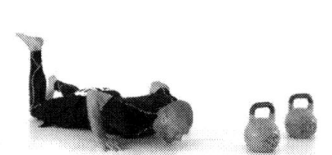 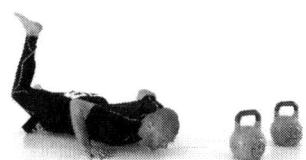

2) Prone thoracic hyperextensions

These are to connect with your erector spinae muscle groups which are to be contracted and simply hold the spine straight (erect) to be moved by the pelvis.

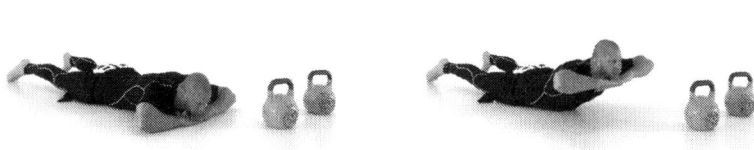

3) Kneeling hip extensions

These are to connect with hamstring muscles which will be pulling at the bottom of your pelvis and help to pull it up during the upswing.

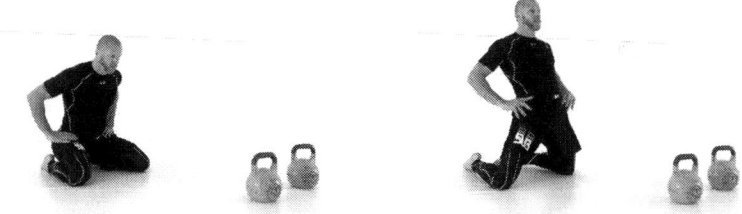

4) Kneeling lunge and pulse

The goals of these is two-fold, the pull with the front leg activates the hamstrings, and the hips coming forward digs into the psoas on the side that the leg is kneeling.

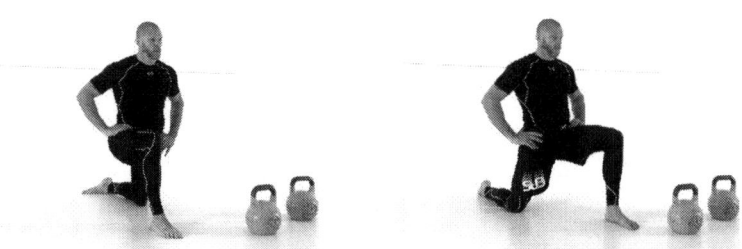

5) True hip hinge

The true hip hinge (AKA stiff-legged hip hinge) prepares you for the primal movement of the kettlebell swing.

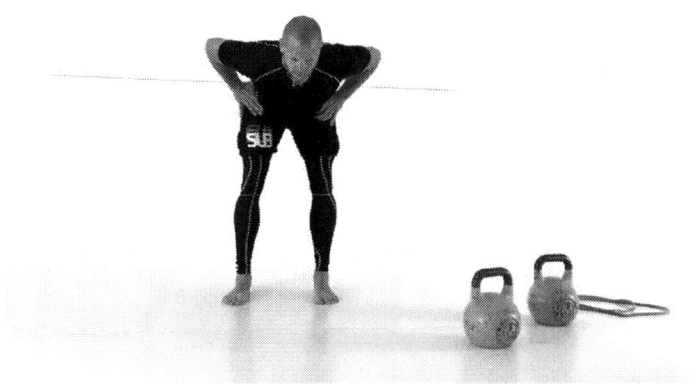

6) Quarter squat

These are to target the quadriceps which are responsible for knee extension which happens at the same time as hip extension.

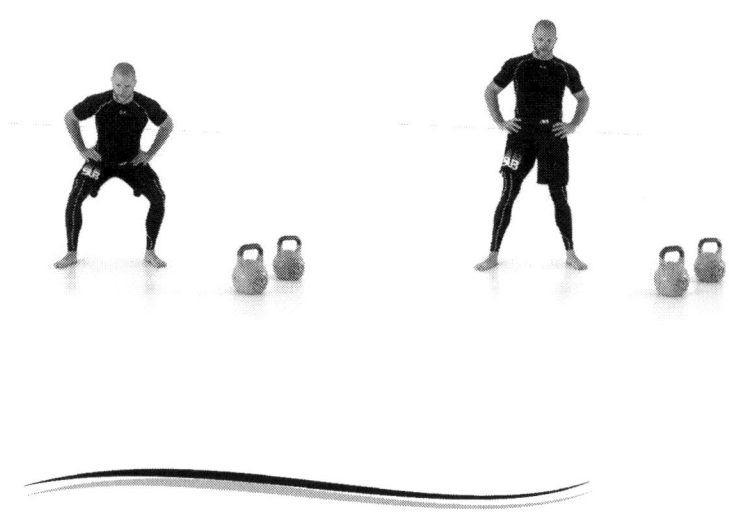

Master The Hip Hinge

Hip Hinge Drills

A great drill to assist with the hip hinge movement is to stand with the back towards the wall, standing just far enough away so that when in the hang phase of the movement the buttocks are touching the wall (for most people, about 20cm/8inch or 30cm/12inch). Now perform the movement, and aim to get the buttocks touching the wall. Focus on bending the knees but keeping them above the ankles (shins vertical).

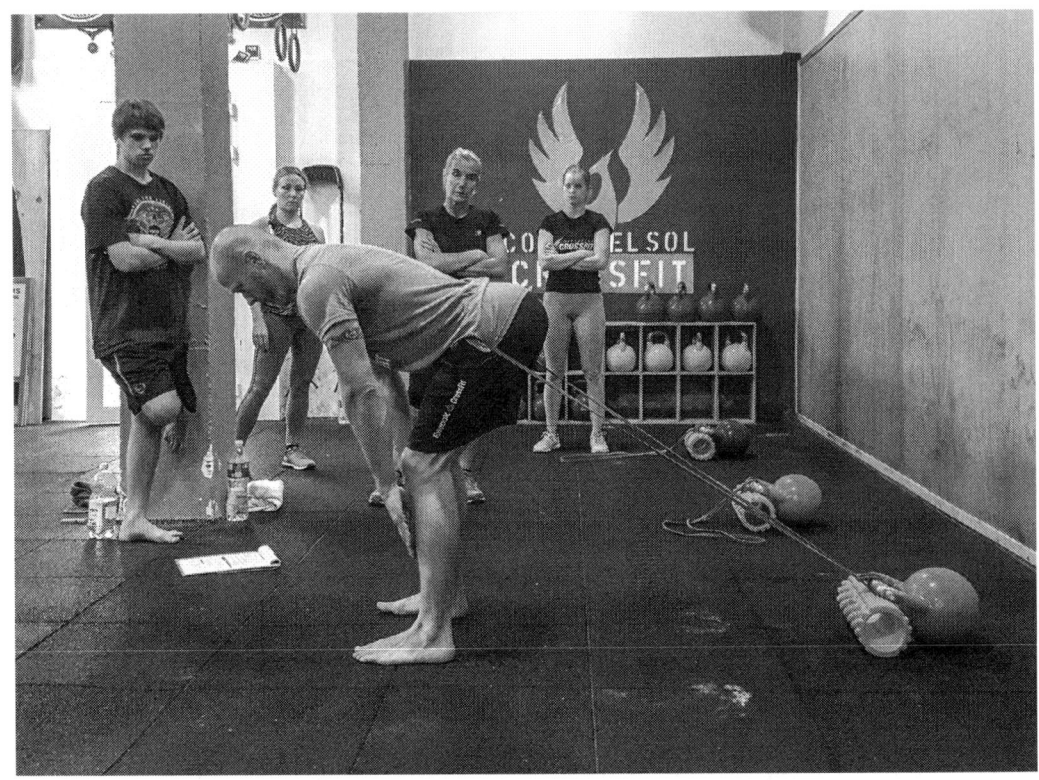

Resistance band drill.

The second drill to assist with the movement is with a resistance band that's anchored low to the ground, which helps create more hip distance going back and down. Due to the position of the anchor, the force is pulling the hips back but also down at the same time. An added bonus is that this drill also provides resistance on the up phase, representing the move that much better.

Corrections

A great way to correct the hip hinge movement is by asking the participant to assume the hang phase of the movement and remain there; this is the point where you provide corrections.

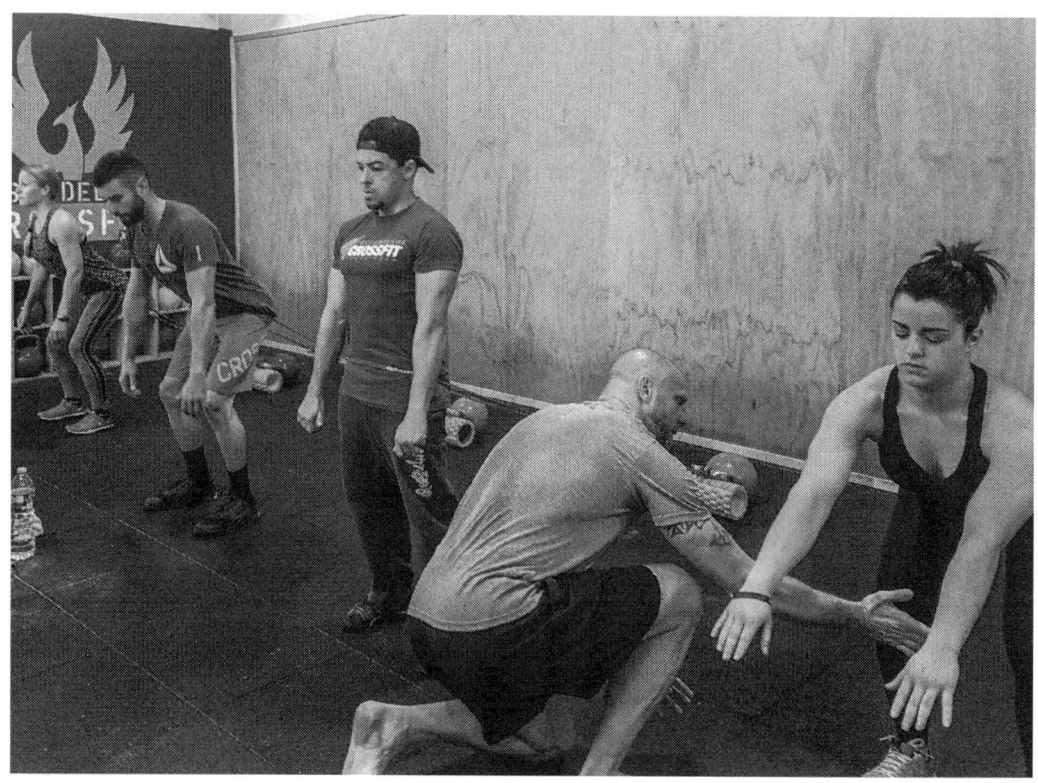

Resistance band drill with corrections.

If the issue is

the participants' knees are forward, torso is not coming down, and the movement resembles more of a squat, the corrections are as follows:

- Ask the participant to move their knees back till they're above the ankles: you can slowly move your hand towards their knees and ask them not to touch your hands.
- Tell them it's ok to feel the stretch at the back of their legs: this is normal and expected.
- To get the hips back, remember the back-to-wall drill.

- Another way to get the hips back is standing in-front and to the side of the participant, and make a pointing movement towards the wall with verbal cues like "hips back more".
- To get the hips down, remember the resistance band with a low anchor drill.
- Another way to get the hips down is by standing in-front and to the side of the participant while making a flat-handed up and down movement towards the ground with verbal cues like "hips down more".
- Ask the participant to do some squats and pay attention to where they're feeling it— if done correctly, they'll be feeling it in the quads (the front of their upper legs); make them understand that this is not where they should be feeling the hip hinge, and if they do, they're probably squatting instead.
- Ask the participant to lower the shoulders towards the ground; you can do this by bringing your flat hand closer to the persons face and then ask them to follow it downwards while keeping the hips at the height they are.

If the issue is

the participants' back is rounded rather than neutral, the corrections are as follows:

- Ask the participant to push out their bellybutton followed by their spine.
- Ask the participant to push out their chest and bring their shoulders back.

All of the above corrections can also be demonstrated side-on and in front of the participant paired with verbal cues. Showing the participant the incorrect position they're in through demonstration and correction is also extremely effective.

Once you have the participant in the correct position, you should make it clear to them that this is the position they need to work towards. If the participant is a novice, it's more than likely they won't yet be able to achieve that position on every repetition—this is due to either, muscle weakness, tightness, unawareness, or simply not used to the movement yet. Typically, however, good form becomes a habit within the first few weeks.

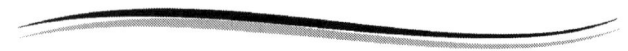

Back Aches and Pains

The majority of freely available research on the Internet—if not all—will tell you that if you experience lower back pain, you're using your back to lift rather than your glutes and legs. This is great information, but it does not exactly tell you why or what the cause is.

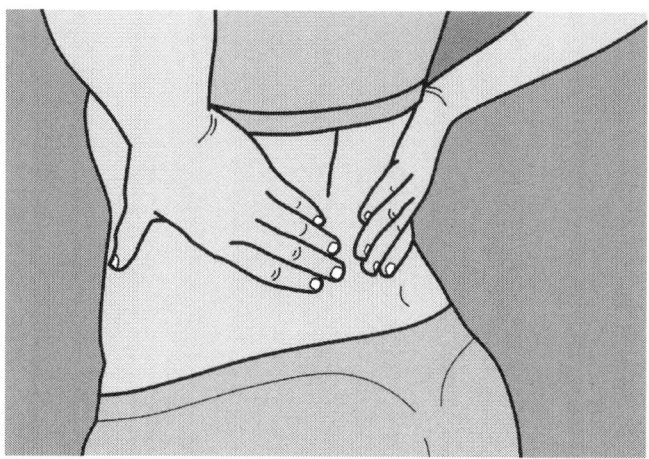

What does it mean to "lift with your back"? It's hard to understand what lifting with your back means without proper explanation, so I'm going to break it down for you in order for you to better understand exactly why your back may hurt after hip hinging, whether for deadlifts, rows, or kettlebell swings.

First you need to understand the key muscles involved: I've listed all of them previously, but I'm going to recap for the explanation of lower-back pain specifically.

The erector spinae, AKA spinal erectors, is a set of muscle groups that straighten and rotate the back. The groups consist of the Iliocostalis, Longissimus and Spinalis.

The Iliocostalis consists of the Iliocostalis Cervicis (which is located near the neck), Iliocostalis Thoracis (which is located near the upper- middle-back), and most importantly the **Iliocostalis Lomborum** which is located near the Lumbar or lower back; this last one will be our focus from this group.

The Longissimus consists of the Longissimus Capitis (which is located near the head),

Longissimus Cervicis (which is located near the neck), and finally the **Longissimus Thoracis** which is located near the middle- lower-back; again, this last one will be our focus from this group, and some more details will be provided on this muscle, such as insertion and origin.

The Spinalis consists of the Spinalis Cervicis (which is located near the neck), and **Spinalis Thoracis,** which is located near the lower-back—this last one will be our focus from this group.

To understand where the above muscles are connected (origin and insertion) to the spine, please review the following illustration of the human spine. Anything with C is the Cervical area, T is the Thoracic and L is the Lumbar region of the spine.

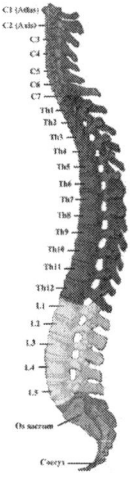

The Quadratus Lumborum is another important muscle group in the lower back. Because the Quadratus Lumborum connects the pelvis to the spine, and is therefore capable of extending the lower back when contracting bilaterally, these two muscles can pick up the slack, as it were, when the lower fibers of the erector spinae are weak or inhibited.

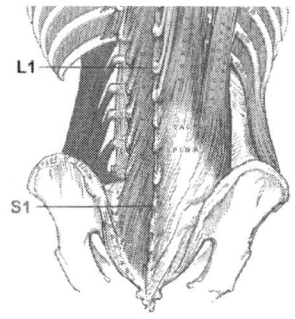

As mentioned earlier, the focus is on forms of lower back pain, therefore we will focus on the following muscles; Iliocostalis Lomborum, Longissimus Thoracis, Spinalis Thoracis and Quadratus Lumborum. On a side note, all of these muscles are bilateral (i.e. are located on both the left and right sides of the body).

1. The Iliocostalis Lomborum **origin** is the sacrum, and the **insertion** is on the first half of the ribs.
2. The Longissimus Thoracis **origin** is around the sacrum and lumbar, and the **insertion(s)** are on all the ribs.
3. The Quadratus Lumborum **origin** is around the top of the pelvis, and the **insertion** is around L1 to L4 and half of the 12th rib.
4. The Spinalis Thoracis **origin** is around the lumbar or thoracic area, and the **insertion** is at the thoracic area.

To summarize, the collective origin of the first three is the lower back, and with insertion from the first rib up. Therefore these three are the most likely to be affected when lifting with the back rather then the hips/legs. By contrast the fourth will more than likely be affected when lifting with the upper back.

To understand one of the major causes for lower back pain, I'm going to ask you to remember the muscles that actually erect the back, visualize all this together with the spine, pelvis and the gluteus maximus.

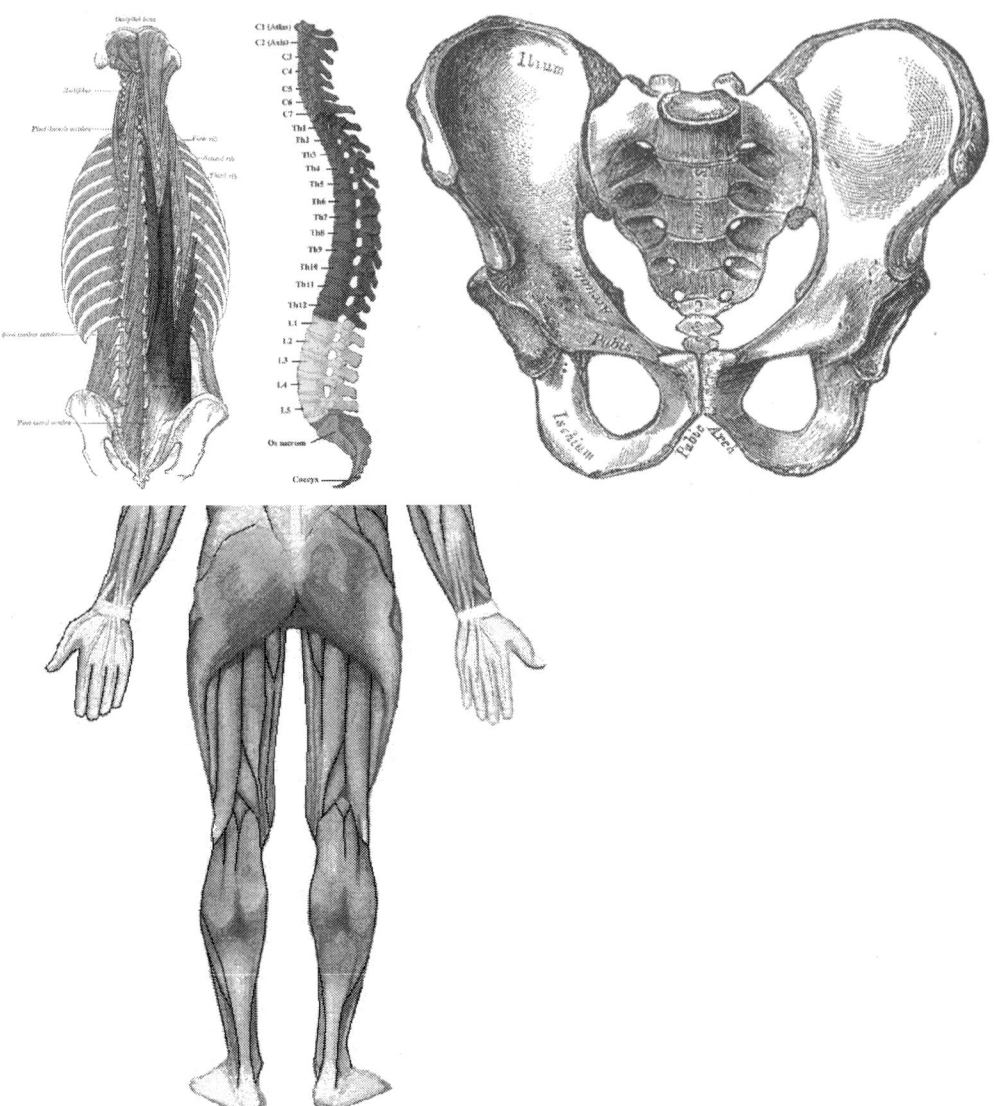

Next, I'm going to ask you to perform a few drills to physically feel and better understand the explanation that follows.

- Come into the hang phase of the hip hinge and remain there, i.e. static hip hinge.
- Find the top of your hip bones (Ilium) with your thumbs; leave the thumbs there.
- Find the top of your femur (thigh bone) with your index fingers; leave the fingers there.
- The location of your thumbs and fingers will give you a general indication of the angle of your pelvis.

- Leave your pelvis in the same position while your back comes up about an inch and towards the starting position.
- Repeat this several times until you feel what muscles are doing the work, which should be your lower back muscles. You could get the one-inch movement with just the upper back (thoracic), but focus on the lower part, the area in which you've (possibly) experienced back pain before.
- Now that you've connected with the muscles of the lower back, we're going to come fully upright while having the lower back muscles do the work, meaning they're *leading*...
- The pelvis will naturally **follow,** as a full upright position is not possible without the pelvis returning into neutral position.
- Repeat this five or so times with a safe, controlled pace, focussing on the feeling, the muscles activated, and on what muscles are leading.
- Now imagine yourself on a steel crane with a powerful engine—your pelvis is the crane and your gluteus maximus are the engine.
- You know the engine can lift a heavy weight with ease, but you're going to try and pull the crane up with your own strength rather than relying on the engine.
- This is exactly what you've been doing in the first phase of this drill; you were not using the powerful engine that is specifically designed to pull the weight up, instead using your back.
- Next you're coming back into a static hip hinge.
- You're going to activate your abdominal and back muscles to create a solid steel crane out of your pelvis and spine. Your abdominal and back muscles are going to be the support for the crane by just holding it upright, nothing else.
- Now you're going to turn your engine on by activating your gluteus maximus, if you need to, you will kick your engine a few times (hit yourself in the gluteus) to get it going.
- Now you're going to connect with your hamstrings, if you need to connect with them, lift your heel to your hips on both sides a few times .
- You're going to come upright by letting the hip extensors move the pelvis first, and have the spine/back follow, *not* lead.

If you do all this right and still experience lower back pain, it's time to ask yourself: did your engine run out of fuel, and require you to pull the weight up by hand? If you're doing everything right but too many repetitions of an exercise, or using a weight that's too heavy, then your engine (hip extensors) might require help from external sources (your weaker back muscles). Build yourself up.

Your back muscles will always need to do work, but the work should be that of creating a steel crane to hold the weight—nothing more—, and the hip extensors should do the work of hoisting the weight. Whether you're deadlifting, barbell cleaning, or swinging a kettlebell, your pelvis should move first and remain the moving hinge upon which your spine is simply moving along, never leading.

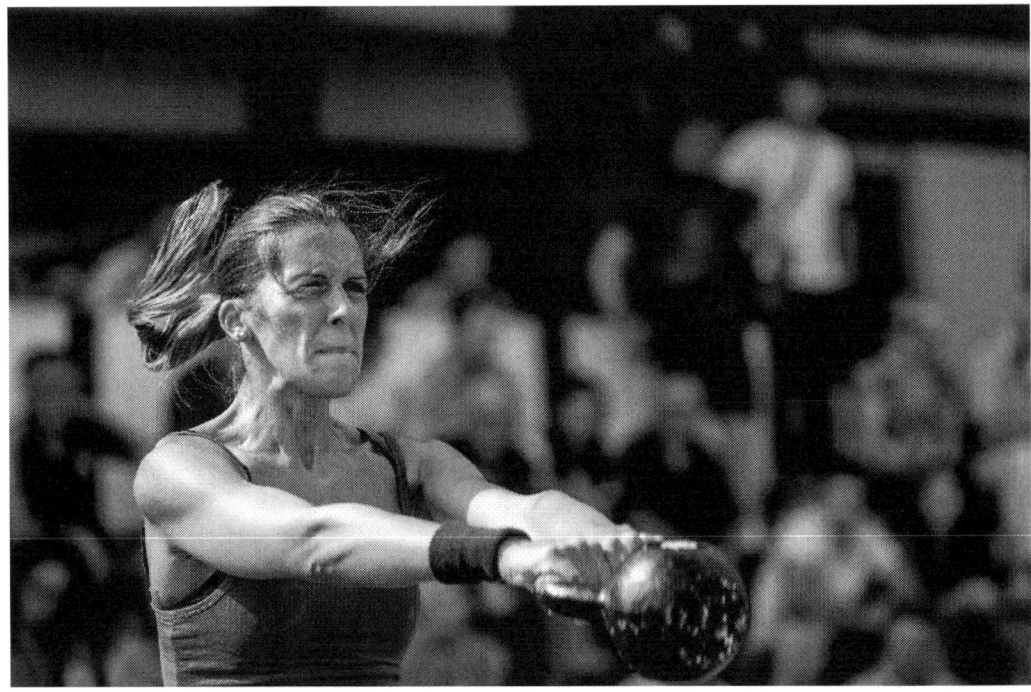

Another important part of preventing pain and injuries is proper pelvic alignment during the hip hinge movement, especially weighted hip hinges. Remember that the spine is positioned upon the pelvis, thus correct alignment between the pelvis and the lumbar is important for proper posture and support of weight. The pelvis can have excessive anterior or posterior tilt, lateral tilt is also possible, but that's a rare exception due to scoliosis or one leg shorter than the other. There are other adverse conditions that cause back pain—like bulging or slipped discs—but in the majority of cases, the cause is simply lifting too heavy or incorrect technique.

In the case of the hip hinge, one should focus on keeping the pelvis aligned with the spine. If the torso comes down, the pelvis should come along through contraction of the hip flexors; once maximum pelvic range is reached, a safe maximum depth has been reached and no further depth should be created with spinal flexion. On the up phase, the pelvis should lead through contraction of the hip extensors.

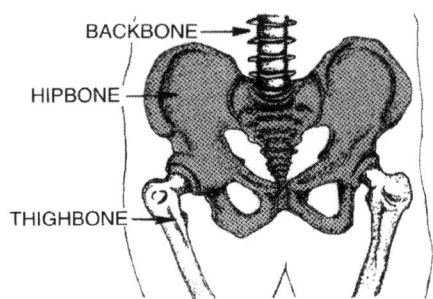

On the down phase you want to avoid posterior pelvic tilt and keep pulling the top of the pelvis down to maintain a neutral position. On the up phase you want to avoid anterior pelvic tilt and keep pulling the top of the pelvis up to maintain a neutral position, but most importantly, at all times avoiding excessive tilt of the pelvis in either direction.

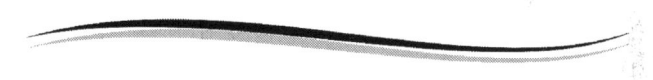

Supercharge Your Weightlifting

Now is a good time to talk about how you can supercharge your weightlifting by using hip hinges with powerful leg drive. Just like you create a steel beam around your spine, you can create a more solid structure that drives into the ground rather than just standing there and carrying weight; you do this by actively driving your heels into the ground.

To become strong on many major lifts—but especially the hip hinge—it's important to drive your heels into the ground, the structure right under your support beams (legs). Yes, you can also spread your toes and push the balls of your feet into the ground to add to the support and drive, but it's important to not have the majority of the drive come from there and nearly none at the heel.

The second reason you want to push your feet into the ground is to create a pushing action from the bottom half of your body, which lightens the pulling action required. Pushing into the ground could also mean the initial lift off, no matter how small, it can create the momentum required to finish the pull, especially with heavy weight.

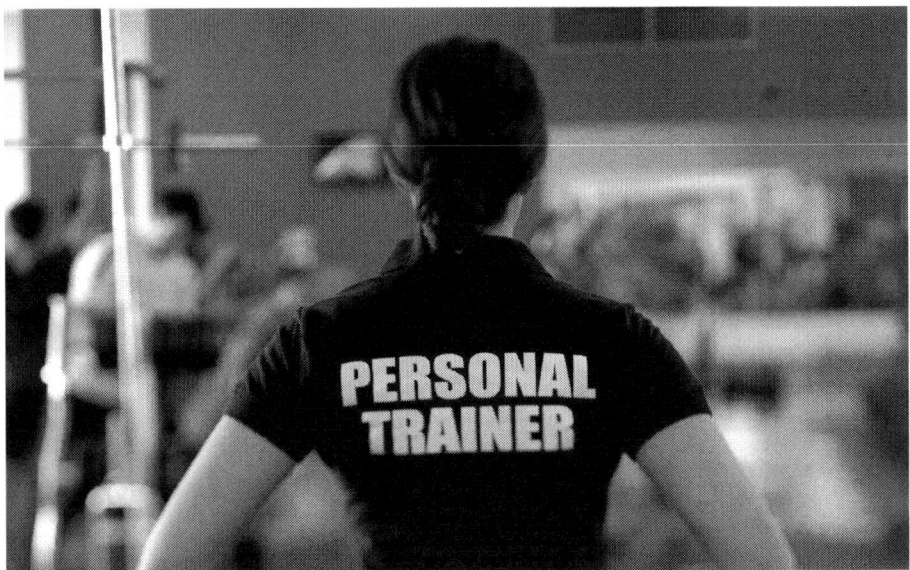

Cues

Following are some cues that will help if you're a Trainer:

- Head in line with the torso

- Neutral head alignment

- Shoulders back, chest out

- Arms relaxed

- Gluteus maximus contracted

- Squeeze the glutes

- Active core

- Abs braced

- Feeling tension on the hamstrings

- Knees bend, but not coming forward

- Knees in line with the ankles

- Shins vertical

- Weight evenly distributed

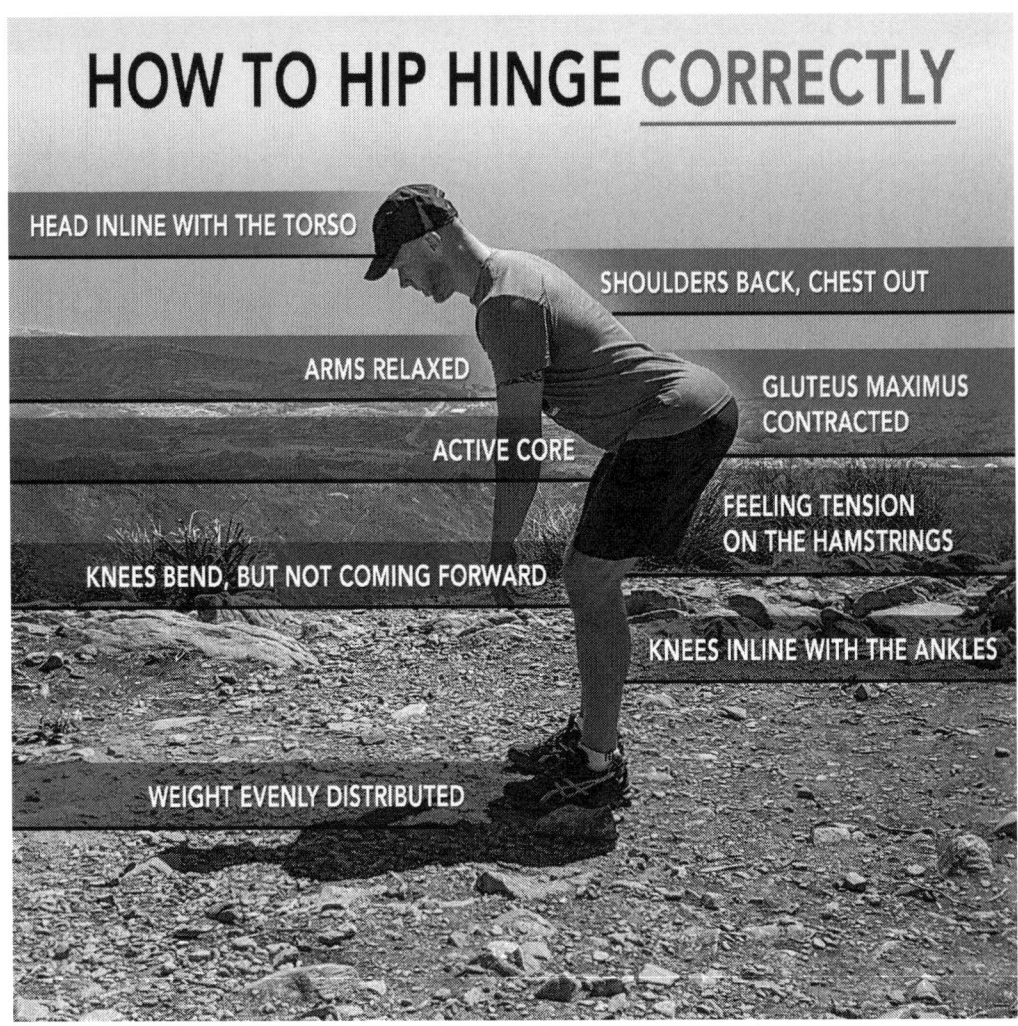

Feel free to share this infographic on Facebook

facebook.com/groups/kettlebell.swing/permalink/643112396076562/

What is "Pulling Yourself Down"?

First, let's list how most downward movements can be executed by the body:

1. Controlled descent

2. Falling descent

3. Pulling descent

In the case of the hip hinge, a **controlled descent** would be where the torso comes forward and down towards the ground, with the hip extensors controlling the speed of descent through slowly relaxing the muscle.

A **falling descent** is when no muscles control the descent until reaching bottom position, and where the muscles stop the descent through a sudden contraction.

For a **pulling descent**, the hip extensors are activated to control the descent, and the hip flexors pull the torso down toward the bottom position through contraction. Both the anterior and posterior muscles are at work.

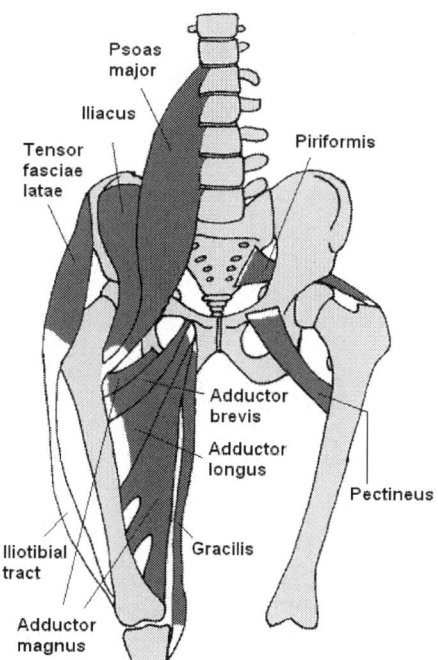

Master The Hip Hinge   *Author Taco Fleur*

The Movement

Following describes the movement for the stiff legged hip hinge step by step, the same principle with slight adjustments applies to most hip hinge variations:

1. Stand in upright neutral stance—neutral phase
2. Initiate flexion with the hip flexors—down phase
3. Pull yourself down
4. Follow with a braced spine
5. Control decent with the hip extensors
6. Maximum range is when the pelvis does not move forward any further
7. Do not create a range with the spine
8. Keep pulling till the maximum range has been reached—hang phase
9. Initiate extension with the hip extensors—up phase
10. Press the heels into the ground to activate the hamstrings
11. Contract the glutes
12. Follow with a braced spine
13. Continue both contractions till the neutral phase has been achieved

Don't Fall Into a Hinge

It's so easy to get lazy with with the down phase of the hip hinge, stay focussed and contract the hip flexors. Use the hip extensors to control the decent. Falling descents are prone to injury due to lack of muscle control during the fast movement.

Hip Hinge Variations

There are five variations to the hip hinge movement pattern;

1. **The straight-legged hip hinge** is performed by keeping the knees locked out;

and only the torso comes forward and down; this is purest form of a hip hinge

2. **The conventional hip hinge** is performed with the knees bent; the hips move slightly back and down while the torso comes forward and down; this is the most known variation of the hip hinge

3. **The staggered hip hinge** is the conventional hip hinge performed with one leg positioned back and approx. 45 degrees out to the side

4. **The conventional one-legged hip hinge** is the same as number 2 but performed with one leg on the ground, and the other coming up at the rear while remaining locked out or bent

5. **The straight one-legged hip hinge** is the same as number 1 but performed with one leg on the ground, and the other coming up at the rear while remaining locked out or bend

You Tube   Watch the video to see some of the variations (including incorrect technique) in action go.cavemantraining.com/mthh-vid8

The straight-legged hip hinge is also called the stiff legged hip hinge, it should be noted that when resistance is added to the exercise, the hips will be moving slightly backwards to prevent falling forward. However, with bodyweight only, it's quite possible to keep the hips above the ankles. Whether to lock the knees out or not is a highly debated topic, I do not recommend locking the knees out when lifting extremely heavy.

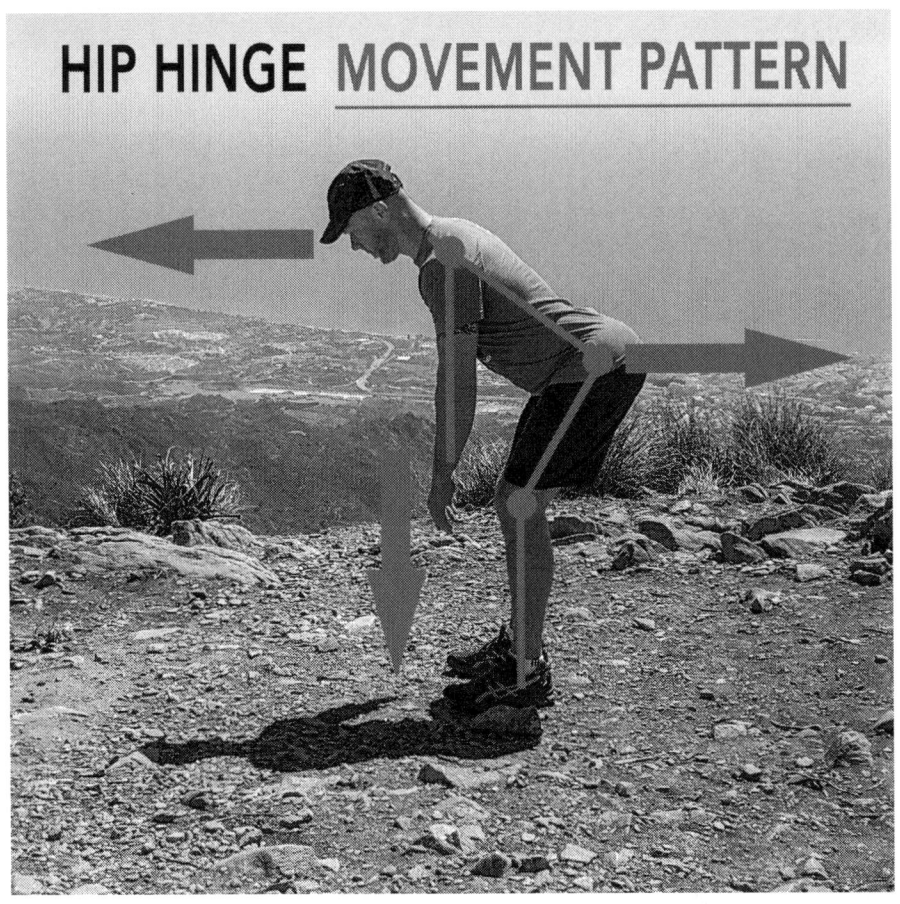

HIP HINGE MOVEMENT PATTERN

Feel free to share this infographic on Facebook

facebook.com/groups/kettebells.for.beginners/permalink/1364097177022718/

Conventional Hip Hinge

The conventional hip hinge movement is performed by following these steps:

- Stand straight.

- Feet placed approximately under the hips/shoulders.

- Chest slightly out.

- Let the arms hang.

- Engage the core muscles; abdominals flexed like someone is going to punch you in the stomach.

- Initiate the movement with the hips by pulling the top of the pelvis down with the hip flexors (front).

- Flex your hip extensors to control the movement (back).

- Your knees are bending but not moving forward; the knees remain in line with the ankles.

- As you're pulling yourself down further toward the ground you will feel a bigger stretch in the hamstrings.

- Your hips will be moving back and down as you come more towards the ground.

- Your back should never round—maintain a neutral spine; If your back starts to round it will more than likely be due to having reached the maximum depth with your hamstring flexibility; Do not go any further.

- Keep your shoulders back and chest out.

- Your head is preferably aligned with your torso, i.e. it follows you as you come down, you can choose to slightly tilt your head backwards if this helps you keep your shoulders back and chest out, but don't strain the neck.

- Come back up by pushing the feet into the ground and contracting the hip extensors.

- Similar to the down phase of this movement, you initiate the up phase by pulling the pelvis up.

![YouTube] Watch the video online to see this movement in action go.cavemantraining.com/mthh-vid1 or with a 32kg kettlebell go.cavemantraining.com/mthh-vid2

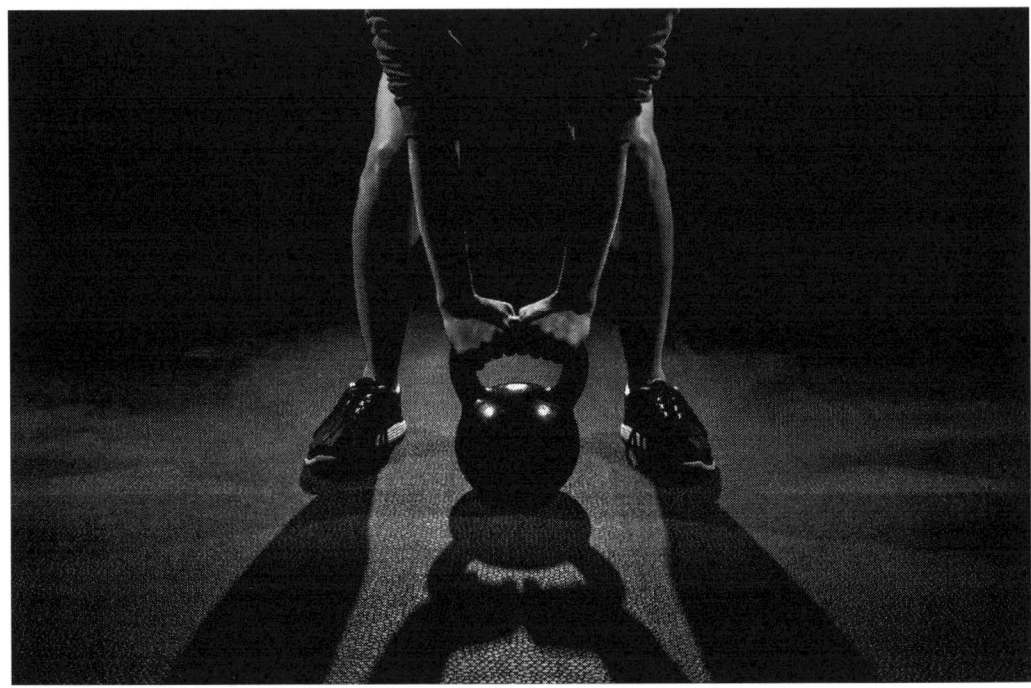

Straight-Legged Hip Hinge

This movement has the following differences from the conventional hip hinge: the legs stay straight; the hips move slightly back but not down by action from the top of the femur moving back to create counterbalance. More hamstring flexibility is required for this movement.

Conventional One-Legged Hip Hinge

This movement has the following differences from the conventional hip hinge: one leg is raised to the rear, in line with the torso; more stability is required; and more strength is required, as only one side of the hip extensors are doing the work.

Straight One-Legged Hip Hinge

This movement has the following differences from the straight-legged hip hinge: one leg is raised to the rear, inline with the torso; more stability is required; more flexibility is required; and more strength is required, as only one side of the hip extensors are doing the work.

Staggered Hip Hinge

The staggered hip hinge is a great way to progress to the one-legged hip hinge. This movement is similar to the one-legged conventional hip hinge. The objective is to take one leg out of the equation, but still provide some assistance and stabilization by keeping the ball of the foot on the ground in a staggered stance.

Throughout any of the movements it is important to keep any added weight evenly distributed. You'll feel when it becomes uneven by when your feet are shifting one way or the other.

If this movement is performed correctly, the arms will only move down and not forward when looking at the movement side on.

Incorrect Muscle Engagement

It should be noted that this movement can also—**incorrectly**—be performed by not engaging the right muscles. For example, one can simply let the body fall forward without pulling it forward and controlling the down phase. The movement can be initiated by the erector spinae and the lower back is doing the work on the up phase, as covered earlier.

You▶️ Watch the video to see the falling descent and other incorrect techniques

Master The Hip Hinge *Author **Taco Fleur***

Common mistakes

- Bending forward on the down phase instead of folding at the hips. This means the shoulders come forward **before** hip flexion.

- Knees coming forward and turning this movement into a squat, which also brings more focus on the anterior chain rather than keeping the focus on the posterior chain muscles.

- Bringing the torso up first by using the erector spinae (your back) to come up, which will affect the back, can cause injury and pain because there is little or no hip drive, i.e. hip extension is not created first. Watch this video to see lifting with the back go.cavemantraining.com/mthh-vid4

- Creating range with the spine, this means that the pelvis has reached maximum range, and further range is created through lowering the shoulders to the ground, i.e. bending the spine (spinal flexion).

Rounding Back

A rounding back is a very common mistake seen with beginners, hence, I will cover it here. The rounding of the back happens because maximum range of hip flexion (pulling the top of the pelvis forward) has been reached, the hamstrings stretch no further, and the subject will want to create more range through thoracic flexion, i.e. creating range with the spine. This is incorrect and not the objective of a hip hinge.

Hip Mobility

Following are some great drills, exercises and stretches to improve hip mobility:

Lying hip rotations

- Lay flat on your back
- Both knees bend
- Feet flat on the ground
- Bring the foot of the active leg over the other knee
- Keep the foot positioned over the other knee throughout this exercise
- The knee of the active leg is pointing laterally outwards
- Create movement in the active leg by bringing the knee towards the chest and back
- Perform this movement without resistance 3 times or more
- Then add resistance by gently pushing the knee of the active leg further away with your hand
- Repeat the full sequence 5 to 10 times on each leg
- Hold the stretch a bit longer as you're going up in reps

If the stretch is not effective, i.e. you do not feel the muscle stretching, then bring the knee of the inactive leg closer to you by bringing the heel closer to your buttocks. You can also grab the knee with the arm on the same side and pull the knee more towards you, increasing the stretch.

https://go.cavemantraining.com/mthh-vid5
Around the 20-second mark you can see me perform a shinbox getup—this exercise is amazing to promote hip mobility. In the same video you'll see me do other variations of getups; they all promote hip mobility. You can do them with or without resistance.

https://go.cavemantraining.com/mthh-vid6
Around the 26-second mark you can see me sitting back; this is great for hip mobility, try rocking back and forth like this yourself, you can also put your shins and feet flat on the ground if you're not going into a plank position.

https://go.cavemantraining.com/mthh-link1
Check out the above article which also comes paired with a video demonstrating many movements, positions, and stretches you can perform while watching TV.

Master The Hip Hinge   *Author Taco Fleur*

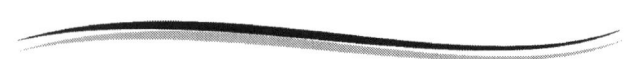

Thank You

Thank you for your purchase of this book. This book is continuously updated with added information. To receive a **free copy of updated versions** in the future please leave your email on the following link http://eepurl.com/dfC-8L.

Become certified

Show your knowledge and become a certified Caveman Trainer online in pressing, swinging or other areas. Visit cavemantraining.com for up-to-date courses or certification online.

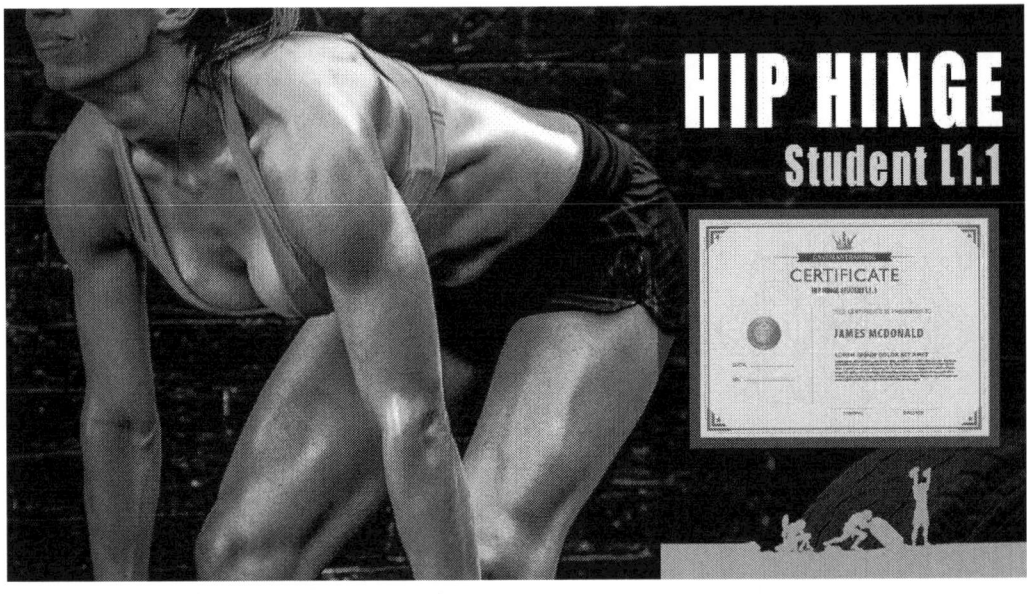

Want to learn a new workout each week?

Join the Caveman Inner Circle where a select group of people from across the world complete one of the Cavemantraining workouts together. Not only do you get access to a unique workout each week, you also get access to two kettlebell coaches, and each workout has a progression or alternative, meaning anyone can do them.

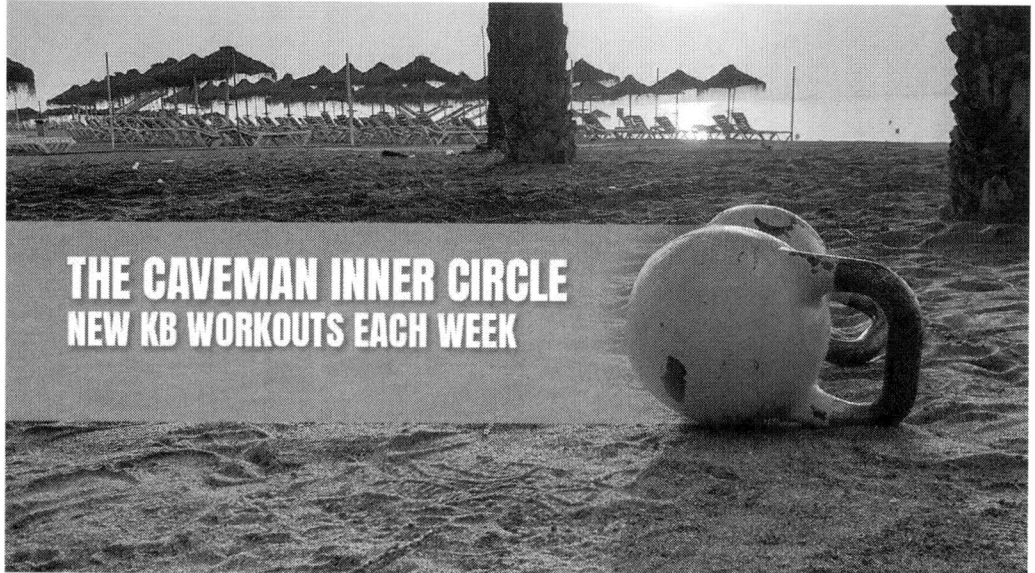

What do you think? Seriously! What do you think?

I want your feedback about this book, was it what you expected, did it not meet your expectations, did you see any areas that can be improved? I love to hear from you, if it's negative feedback, please accompany it with constructive feedback, if you have positive feedback, please consider leaving a review below or on Amazon:

www.facebook.com/pg/caveman.training/reviews/

info@cavemantraining.com

me@tacofleur.com

www.facebook.com/taco.fleur

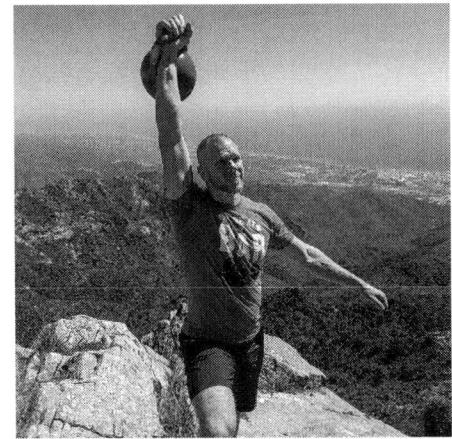

Check out the Cavemantraining channel http://bit.ly/25pqCfA

www.youtube.com/Cavemantraining

Written by Taco Fleur

Copyright owned by Taco Fleur and Cavemantraining

www.cavemantraining.com

THANKS

Big thanks to the following people for helping make this book happen.

Sean Wells from Solid State Fitness for helping tidy up the grammar and spelling.

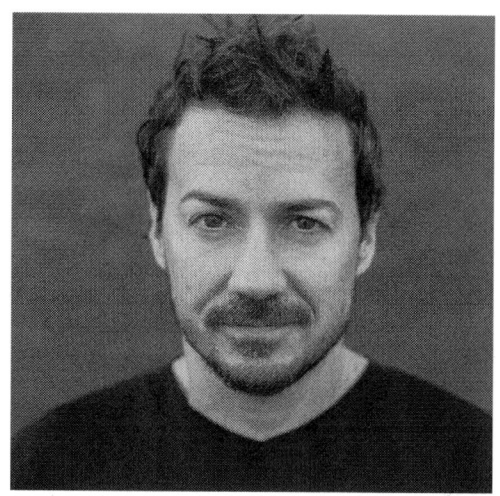

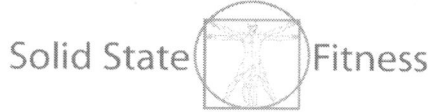

With the help from
Wendy Chappell, Tony Gomez, Anna Junghans, Benooi Fleur Junghans and Derek Fronczak

www.cavemantraining.com

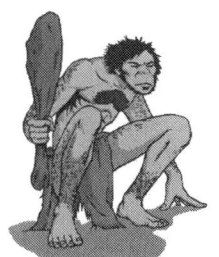
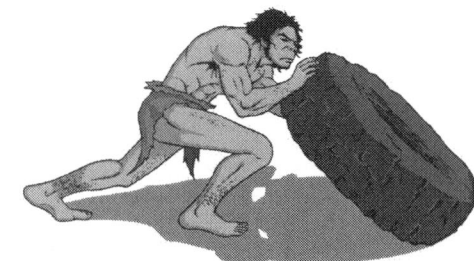
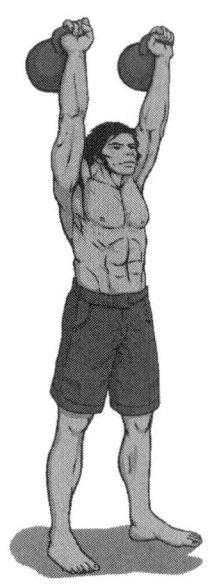

Master The Hip Hinge

Author Taco Fleur